CANCER AND COMPLEMENTARY MEDICINE: *Your Guide to Smart Choices in Symptom Management*

By
Colleen O. Lee, MS, CRNP, AOCN®, CLNC
Georgia M. Decker, APRN, ANP-BC, CN®, AOCN®

ONS Publications Department
Executive Director, Professional Practice and Programs:
Elizabeth M. Wertz Evans, RN, MPM, CPHQ, CPHIMS, FACMPE
Publisher and Director of Publications: Barbara Sigler, RN, MNEd
Managing Editor: Lisa M. George, BA
Technical Content Editor: Angela D. Klimaszewski, RN, MSN
Staff Editor II: Amy Nicoletti, BA
Copy Editor: Laura Pinchot, BA
Graphic Designer: Dany Sjoen

Library of Congress Cataloging-in-Publication Data

Lee, Colleen O.
    Cancer and complementary medicine : your guide to smart choices in symptom management / by Colleen O. Lee and Georgia M. Decker.
        p. cm.
    Includes bibliographical references.
    ISBN 978-1-935864-17-2 (alk. paper)
    1. Cancer--Alternative treatment. I. Decker, Georgia M. II. Title.
    RC271.A62L44 2012
    616.99'4--dc23

                                                              2012006583

Publisher's Note

This book is published by the Oncology Nursing Society (ONS). ONS neither represents nor guarantees that the practices described herein will, if followed, ensure safe and effective patient care. The recommendations contained in this book reflect ONS's judgment regarding the state of general knowledge and practice in the field as of the date of publication. The recommendations may not be appropriate for use in all circumstances. Those who use this book should make their own determinations regarding specific safe and appropriate patient-care practices, taking into account the personnel, equipment, and practices available at the hospital or other facility at which they are located. The editors and publisher cannot be held responsible for any liability incurred as a consequence from the use or application of any of the contents of this book. Figures and tables are used as examples only. They are not meant to be all-inclusive, nor do they represent endorsement of any particular institution by ONS. Mention of specific products and opinions related to those products do not indicate or imply endorsement by ONS. Web sites mentioned are provided for information only; the hosts are responsible for their own content and availability. Unless otherwise indicated, dollar amounts reflect U.S. dollars.

ONS publications are originally published in English. Publishers wishing to translate ONS publications must contact ONS about licensing arrangements. ONS publications cannot be translated without obtaining written permission from ONS. (Individual tables and figures that are reprinted or adapted require additional permission from the original source.) Because translations from English may not always be accurate or precise, ONS disclaims any responsibility for inaccuracies in words or meaning that may occur as a result of the translation. Readers relying on precise information should check the original English version.

Printed in the United States of America

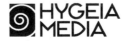

An imprint of the Oncology Nursing Society

CONTENTS

DISCLOSURE

Editors and authors of books and guidelines provided by the Oncology Nursing Society are expected to disclose to the readers any significant financial interest or other relationships with the manufacturer(s) of any commercial products.

A vested interest may be considered to exist if a contributor is affiliated with or has a financial interest in commercial organizations that may have a direct or indirect interest in the subject matter. A "financial interest" may include, but is not limited to, being a shareholder in the organization; being an employee of the commercial organization; serving on an organization's speakers bureau; or receiving research from the organization. An "affiliation" may be holding a position on an advisory board or some other role of benefit to the commercial organization. Vested interest statements appear in the front matter for each publication.

Contributors are expected to disclose any unlabeled or investigational use of products discussed in their content. This information is acknowledged solely for the information of the readers.

The author provided the following disclosure and vested interest information:

Georgia M. Decker, APRN, ANP-BC, CN®, AOCN®: ONS:Edge, Board of Directors; American Cancer Society Great Lakes Division, honoraria

CHAPTER 1

WHAT IS COMPLEMENTARY AND ALTERNATIVE MEDICINE, AND CAN IT BE USED SAFELY?

INTRODUCTION

C ancer often harms a person's physical, mental, and emotional well-being, and the treatments, such as chemotherapy, radiation, and surgery, can be just as devastating. People with cancer are all too familiar with these effects: anxiety, depression, fatigue, nausea and vomiting, pain, sleep disturbances, to list just a few. Dealing with these effects can take a toll on patients, leading many to look to alternatives. *Complementary and alternative medicine*, or CAM, has become widely used among people with cancer seeking relief from these symptoms and side effects. But this increased use comes with many questions. The purpose of this book is to give you an introduction to CAM and its use in cancer symptom management. We will examine many different therapies that are being used by people with cancer and will provide information on symptom management, drug interactions and contraindications, CAM use by cancer site, and general health and wellness.

With the distressing effects of cancer and its treatment, it is tempting to want to try anything and everything touted as a "cure" for a particular symptom or ailment you are experiencing. However, regardless of how "natural" or "safe" they may seem, these products have the potential to harm just as readily as any drug can. Before starting any new therapy or practice, it is important that you talk to your healthcare providers.

Keeping you safe during and after your cancer treatment is a primary aim for this handbook. Although we have learned much about CAM through some ongoing research, many questions remain. Therefore, we have included details on reliable resources so you can stay current on this information.

Experts do not always agree about how safe and effective CAM therapies may be. By becoming an informed consumer and communicating openly with your healthcare providers, you can determine whether CAM is appropriate for use in the management of your health.

WHO USES CAM?

According to national surveys, more than 80% of Americans, and more than half of people with cancer, use some form of CAM. The costs are staggering: $33.9 billion in out-of-pocket spending, according to a recent government survey. With this level of usage, the ability to determine whether a therapy is safe and effective is critical.

WHY DO PEOPLE USE CAM?

The reasons for using CAM are as varied as the types of therapies used. Many people use them to

promote general wellness. Others use these therapies to manage symptoms of a diagnosed condition
or side effects of a medical treatment. CAM therapies may be used to promote comfort and relaxation. And people with cancer often use these therapies to complement their medical therapy or to allow them to be active participants in their cancer
treatment.

CAN THESE THERAPIES INTERFERE WITH CANCER TREATMENT?

Some CAM therapies have the potential to interfere
with cancer treatment such as chemotherapy drugs. In
addition, some may interfere with therapies for other
conditions. Just because something is labeled *natural*
does not mean it is *safe*. Even seemingly harmless "natural" supplements can have strong interactions with medications. More on this topic appears in Chapter 3.

DO I HAVE TO TELL ALL OF MY HEALTHCARE PROVIDERS ABOUT MY CAM USE?

To help keep you safe from negative interactions
or a negative effect on treatment, it is important that
you tell all of your healthcare providers about any
CAM therapies you are using, including herbal products and other supplements.

If any CAM practitioner tells you that the therapy he or she offers is a secret and you should not discuss it with your healthcare providers, be very cau-
tious. Likewise, if a practitioner makes promises about
"cures," talk to your healthcare provider before making any decisions about it.

WHAT SHOULD I TELL MY HEALTHCARE PROVIDERS?

It is important to advise your healthcare providers about any herbs, nutritional supplements, vitamins, teas, poultices, and over-the-counter medications you use, whether regularly or just sometimes. Also, inform them of any methods that you use, such as relaxation, guided imagery, Reiki, healing touch, hypnosis, or meditation, whether regularly or occasionally. Once your cancer treatment has ended, it is still important to tell your healthcare providers about any new interventions or methods you have decided to use.

CHOOSING A CAM PRACTITIONER WISELY

Credentialing and Licensure

A CAM practitioner is an individual who delivers CAM therapies and may have certification or licensure from a state or national program. Being "certified" does not always indicate that the practitioner is licensed. *Licensure* refers to the laws that regulate an occupation. These laws protect against unqualified practitioners using a particular occupational title and define the scope of practice of that occupation. Licensure occurs at the state level, and the scope of practice may vary from state to state. In most states, CAM providers who lack licensure could be viewed as diagnosing, treating, and practicing medicine on patients unlawfully.

Certification is a formal recognition by an accrediting body that a practitioner has met predetermined qualifications such as education, practice hours, and examinations. National certification ensures that a professional's credentials will be recognized in most or all states and that the scope of practice is the same or similar in each state.

Selecting a CAM Practitioner

If you are considering a CAM therapy, start by talking with your primary healthcare provider about any CAM therapies you use now and what you may be interested in using in the future. Your healthcare provider may be able to answer questions or refer you to a reputable CAM practitioner. Also, CAM practitioners can be found through professional organizations. Collect information such as education, experience, and cost. Check with your insurance provider to see which practitioners accept your insurance. Make an appointment to speak to the potential practitioner in person or by telephone. Choose a CAM practitioner based on the person's answers to your questions and your level of comfort during the interview. Explain what you do to manage your health to help ensure coordinated and safe care. Assess the practitioner after your initial treatment visit, weighing what you have been told to expect in terms of therapy outcomes, time, and costs. Tips for talking with your healthcare providers about CAM are available online as part of the "Time to Talk" campaign at http://nccam.nih.gov/timetotalk/forpatients.htm. Examples of CAM practices with educational preparation, licensure, and credentialing criteria appear in Chapter 2.

Finding an Integrative Medicine Center

Over the past few decades, integrative medicine programs have begun to open across the country. Integrative medicine combines treatments from conventional medicine and CAM that have evidence of safety and effectiveness. Integrative medicine programs offer a variety of services and may be freestanding, associated with a network of providers, or part of an academic health center. The Consortium of Academic Health Centers for Integrative Medicine (CAHCIM) represents 50 academic health centers and affiliate institutions in the United States and Canada, most of which offer clinical programs that treat many conditions. If you live near one of these programs, you can contact them directly for information on referrals and clinical services. A list of centers is located at www.imconsortium .org/members/home.html, or you can contact CAHCIM by phone at 612-624-9166.

Also, many cancer centers are beginning to include integrative medicine services in their practice. Check with your local cancer centers and hospitals to see if they offer these services.

FOR MORE INFORMATION

- American Cancer Society, www.cancer.org/Treatment/ TreatmentsandSideEffects/Complementaryand AlternativeMedicine/index, or call 800-227-2345 (or 866-228-4327 for TTY). Information on CAM is also included in the sections on specific cancer sites.
- National Institutes of Health National Center for Complementary and Alternative Medicine, http:// nccam.nih.gov/timetotalk, or call 888-644-6226 (or 866-464-3615 for TTY)
- National Cancer Institute PDQ® Cancer Information Summaries, Complementary and Alternative Medicine, www.cancer.gov/cancertopics/pdq/ cam

- National Cancer Institute Office of Cancer Complementary and Alternative Medicine Health Information for Patients, www.cancer.gov/cam/health_ patients.html, or call 301-435-7980
- Your local cooperative extension and the public service announcement section of your local newspaper for classes on healthy cooking or cooking with herbs

RESOURCES

"Categories of CAM therapies," National Cancer Institute, www.cancer.gov/cam/health_categories.html

"Paying for CAM," National Center for Complementary and Alternative Medicine, http://nccam.nih.gov/health/financial

"Selecting a complementary and alternative medicine practitioner," National Center for Complementary and Alternative Medicine, http://nccam.nih.gov/health/decisions/practitioner.htm

"Time to talk," National Center for Complementary and Alternative Medicine, http://nccam.nih.gov/timetotalk

"What is CAM?" National Center for Complementary and Alternative Medicine, http://nccam.nih.gov/health/whatiscam/#types

"What is integrative medicine?" WebMD, www.webmd.com/a-to-z-guides/features/alternative-medicine-integrative-medicine

"What is the difference between having a license and being certified?" Allied Health Licensing, www.nhanow.com/certifications/why-get-certified/licensing-vs-certification.aspx

CHAPTER 2

TYPES OF COMPLEMENTARY AND ALTERNATIVE THERAPIES

CAM THERAPY CATEGORIES

CAM therapies are typically grouped into several main categories. In this book, we will use the following classifications: alternative medical systems, complex natural products, energy therapies, exercise therapies, manipulative and body-based methods, mind-body interventions, nutritional therapeutics, pharmacologic and biologic treatments, and spiritual therapies. Patients with cancer may explore therapies that fall under any of these categories. Here, we will describe the different categories and provide examples of CAM therapies for each. Therapies marked with an asterisk (*) will be described in more detail later in the chapter.

Alternative Medical Systems

- Description: interventions built upon well-developed systems of theory and practice
- Examples: acupuncture*, Ayurveda, homeopathy*, naturopathy*, traditional Chinese medicine

Complex Natural Products

- Description: assortment of botanicals, extracts of crude natural substances, and unfractionated ex-

tracts from marine organisms used for healing and treatment of disease
- Examples: botanicals, green tea*, shark cartilage

Energy Therapies

- Description: therapies involving the use of energy fields
- Examples: qigong*, Reiki*, therapeutic touch, magnet therapy

Exercise Therapies

- Description: therapies used to improve patterns of bodily movement
- Examples: tai chi, yoga*, dance therapy

Manipulative and Body-Based Methods

- Description: therapies based on manipulation and movement of one or more body parts
- Examples: chiropractic, massage*, osteopathy, reflexology

Mind-Body Interventions

- Description: therapies designed to enhance the mind's capacity to have an effect on bodily function and symptoms
- Examples: aromatherapy*, art therapy, cognitive-behavioral therapy, imagery, mindfulness meditation*

Nutritional Therapeutics

- Description: assortment of nutrients, non-nutrients, bioactive food components, and diets that are used for chemoprevention and treatment
- Examples: antioxidants, macrobiotics*, vitamins

Pharmacologic and Biologic Treatments

- Description: drugs, vaccines, and other biologic interventions that are not yet accepted into conventional medicine and the off-label use of prescription drugs
- Examples: high-dose vitamin C, melatonin, mistletoe*

Spiritual Therapies

- Description: therapies focusing on religious beliefs and feelings including an individual's sense of peace, purpose, connection with others, and beliefs about the meaning of life
- Examples: intercessory prayer, distant healing, and healing services

EXAMPLES OF CAM THERAPIES AND THEIR USE

This next section discusses a number of CAM therapies you may be familiar with. For each, a definition, description of its use, information on practitioners, evidence to support its use, potential side effects, and additional resources are presented.

Acupuncture

What is acupuncture?

LAc—licensed acupuncturist

Dipl.Ac.—Diplomate of Acupuncture

Acupuncture involves the stimulation of anatomic points called *acupoints* on the skin. It is based on the belief that qi (pronounced "chee," also known as vital energy) flows through the body along paths called meridians. Qi is said to affect a person's spiritual, emotional, mental, and physical health. Most commonly, acupuncture involves penetrating the skin with thin, solid, metallic needles that are moved by the hands or by electrical stimulation.

Moxibustion is the application of heat to specific acupoints. Burning small, tightly bound herbs called moxa is sometimes used along with acupuncture.

Who practices acupuncture? What certification, licensure, and education options are available?

A Diplomate of Acupuncture has completed three to four years of education at the master's level in an acupuncture program accredited by the Accreditation Commission for Acupuncture and Oriental Medicine (ACAOM). ACAOM is the only accrediting body recognized by the U.S. Department of Education.

In addition to graduating from an ACAOM-accredited program, a Diplomate of Acupuncture must pass the National Certification Commission for Acupuncture and Oriental Medicine certification examinations in Foundations of Oriental Medicine, Acupuncture, and Biomedicine before practicing.

What is the evidence to support the use of acupuncture in cancer care?

Available scientific evidence does not support acupuncture as an effective treatment for cancer or any other disease.

Acupuncture may relieve chronic pain, postoperative pain, and chemotherapy-related nausea and vomiting. Ongoing studies are reviewing the effectiveness of acupuncture for low back pain, headache, and osteoarthritis of the knee; what happens in the brain during acupuncture; and methods and instruments for improving the quality of research.

What are some potential side effects, cautions, or contraindications?

Acupuncture is generally accepted as safe and effective for use in chronic or postoperative pain and chemotherapy-related nausea and vomiting. Acupuncture should be used with caution in patients with valvular heart disease, bleeding disorders, a systemic or local infection, pain of unknown origin, or in skin regions that have been radiated; those on anticoagulant therapy; and those who are pregnant.

Where can I learn more?

"Acupuncture (PDQ®)," National Cancer Institute, www.cancer .gov/cancertopics/pdq/cam/acupuncture/patient

"Acupuncture," American Cancer Society, www.cancer .org/Treatment/TreatmentsandSideEffects/Complementary andAlternativeMedicine/ManualHealingandPhysicalTouch/ acupuncture

"Acupuncture," MedlinePlus, www.nlm.nih.gov/medlineplus/ acupuncture.html

"Acupuncture: An introduction," National Center for Complementary and Alternative Medicine, http://nccam.nih .gov/health/acupuncture/introduction.htm

Columbia University Medical Center: The Integrative Therapies Program for Children with Cancer, http://integrativetherapies .columbia.edu/research/acup.html

"Moxibustion," American Cancer Society, www.cancer.org /Treatment/TreatmentsandSideEffects/Complementary andAlternativeMedicine/ManualHealingandPhysicalTouch/ moxibustion

Aromatherapy

What is aromatherapy?

RA—registered aromatherapist

CCA—certified clinical aromatherapist

Aromatherapy refers to several therapies that deliver essential oils to the body. Essential oils are mixed with a carrier oil or diluted in alcohol before being applied to the skin, sprayed in the air, or inhaled. Each type of oil has a different chemical structure that affects how it smells, how it is absorbed, and how it is used by the body. Essential oils are very concentrated and evaporate quickly when they come in contact with the air. Massage, healing touch, and Reiki are common means of delivering oils onto the body.

Who practices aromatherapy? What certification, licensure, and education options are available?

Credentialing is available through the National Association for Holistic Aromatherapy. Many trained practitioners incorporate aromatherapy in their practice. These practitioners may be self-taught or may have taken courses on aromatherapy methods.

The Institute of Spiritual Healing and Aromatherapy offers two programs. The first program is a clinical aromatherapy program involving essential oil education as a part of a 300-hour course that qualifies students to sit for the national exam to become a registered aromatherapist. The second is an educational program in healing touch called the Healing Touch Spiritual Ministry Program.

What is the evidence to support the use of aromatherapy in cancer care?

Available scientific evidence does not support aromatherapy as an effective treatment for cancer or any other disease.

Aromatherapy has been studied in the treatment of stress, anxiety, and other health-related conditions in patients with mixed results. Aromatherapy may enhance quality of life in patients with cancer. Some patients receiving aromatherapy have improvement in nausea or pain and lower blood pressure, pulse, and respiratory rates.

A small study of tea tree oil as a topical treatment for antibiotic-resistant bacteria on the skin of hospital patients found that it was as effective as the standard therapy. Antibacterial essential oils may reduce the odor associated with necrotic ulcers.

What are some potential side effects, cautions, or contraindications?

Aromatherapy has very few side effects or risks when used as directed. Some essential oils have been approved as ingredients in food and are generally recognized as safe by the U.S. Food and Drug Administration, within specific limits. Eating large amounts of essential oils is not recommended.

Allergic reactions and skin irritation may occur when essential oils are in contact with the skin for long periods of time. Sun sensitivity may result when citrus or other oils are applied before sun exposure. Lavender and tea tree oils have some hormone-like effects. People who have tumors that need estrogen to grow should avoid using lavender and tea tree oils.

Where can I learn more?

"Aromatherapy," American Cancer Society, www.cancer.org/ Treatment/TreatmentsandSideEffects/Complementaryand AlternativeMedicine/MindBodyandSpirit/aromatherapy

"Aromatherapyandessentialoils(PDQ®)," NationalCancerInstitute, www.cancer.gov/cancertopics/pdq/cam/aromatherapy/ patient/AllPages

"Herbs at a glance: Lavender," National Center for Complementary and Alternative Medicine, http://nccam.nih.gov/health/ lavender/ataglance.htm

Green Tea

What is green tea?

Green tea is a drink made from the steamed and dried leaves of the *Camellia sinensis* plant. Black and oolong teas also come from the *Camellia sinensis* plant. Unlike green tea, though, black tea is made from leaves that have been fermented. Fermentation may lessen the level of antioxidants in the tea. Green tea extracts can be formed into capsules and included in skin products.

What is the evidence to support the use of green tea in cancer care?

Available scientific evidence does not support green tea as an effective treatment for cancer or any other disease.

Green tea and its extracts have been used to prevent and treat some cancers, including breast, skin, and stomach cancers. Laboratory studies suggest that compounds in the tea may help stop new blood vessels from forming and may cut off the supply of blood to cancer cells. At this time, though, the available scientific evidence does not support that green tea can help prevent or treat any specific type of cancer in humans.

Green tea and its extracts are also used for improving mental alertness, aiding in weight loss, lowering cholesterol levels, and protecting skin from sun damage. More studies are needed to determine its effectiveness in these areas.

What are some potential side effects, cautions, or contraindications?

Green tea and its extracts contain caffeine, which may cause insomnia, anxiety, irritability, upset stomach, nausea, diarrhea, or sodium and potassium loss related to its diuretic effect. Green tea also contains small amounts of vitamin K, which may make anticoagulant drugs, such as warfarin, less effective.

Allergic reactions may occur with the use of green tea and its extracts and may include cough, shortness of breath, loss of consciousness, asthma, and anaphylaxis in sensitive individuals.

Where can I learn more?

"Green tea," American Cancer Society, www.cancer.org/ Treatment/TreatmentsandSideEffects/Complementary andAlternativeMedicine/HerbsVitaminsandMinerals/green-tea
"Herbs at a glance: Green tea," National Center for Complementary and Alternative Medicine, http://nccam.nih.gov/health/greentea

Homeopathy

Hom—homeopathic physician

What is homeopathy?

Homeopathy is an alternative medical system that uses diluted substances to prompt the body's self-healing mechanism that is believed to bring about symptom or disease resolution. Homeopathy is based on the idea that if a large dose of a substance can cause a symptom, then very small doses of that same substance will cure the symptom. Remedies are alcohol-based or water-based solutions that contain very small amounts of minerals, plants, animal products, or chemicals.

The "classical" homeopathic approach individualizes treatment for patients through thorough interviews focusing on symptoms and finding effective remedies for these symptoms.

Who are homeopaths? What certification, licensure, and education options are available?

Several homeopathic programs are available in the United States, with curriculums ranging from 10 weeks to three years. The American Medical College of Homeopathy offers a homeopathic practitioner program (three years and 1,104 hours) and a Doctor of Classical Homeopathy program (three years and 4,280 clinical hours). No formal licensure process is currently available.

Many trained practitioners incorporate homeopathic methods in their practice. These practitioners may be self-taught or have taken courses on homeopathic methods.

What is the evidence to support the use of homeopathy in cancer care?

Available scientific evidence does not support homeopathy as an effective treatment for cancer or any other disease.

In a small group of patients with cancer who used a homeopathic approach with conventional/traditional therapies, homeopathy decreased reported levels of fatigue and improved quality of life.

Another study showed that Traumeel S®, a homeopathic remedy, decreased the severity of mucositis in children receiving a bone marrow transplant.

What are some potential side effects, cautions, or contraindications?

Limited safety research is available because therapies are often individualized. There are no published reports of serious adverse effects.

Where can I learn more?

American Medical College of Homeopathy, www.amcofh.org

"Homeopathy," American Cancer Society, www.cancer.org/Treatment/TreatmentsandSideEffects/Complementary andAlternativeMedicine/PharmacologicalandBiological Treatment/homeopathy

"Homeopathy: An introduction," National Center for Complementary and Alternative Medicine, http://nccam.nih.gov/health/homeopathy

Macrobiotics
What is macrobiotics?

Macrobiotics is a life approach in addition to a nutritional/diet program. Macrobiotics involves "living simply" with a spiritual, physical, and communal discipline. An important goal of a macrobiotic diet is to balance two energy forms (yin and yang) that followers believe are present within people, food, and objects in order to achieve health and vitality.

Those who practice macrobiotics believe that food and its quality affect health, well-being, and happiness. The nutritional diet is mostly vegetarian with an emphasis on fruits, beans, and seaweeds, with a small amount of white meat or fish once or twice weekly. The three types of macrobiotics are Zen, American, and Integrative Macrobiotics.

Who practices macrobiotics? What certification, licensure, and education options are available?

Several macrobiotic training programs in the United States involve online study and in-person training. Certification requires six months of learning with a focus on caregiver cooking, healthy lifestyle cooking, or becoming a cooking teacher. No formal credentialing or licensure process is currently available. Certification is offered through Macrobiotics America and the Kushi Institute. Many trained practitioners incorporate macrobiotics in their practice.

What is the evidence to support macrobiotic approaches in cancer care?

Available scientific evidence does not support macrobiotics as an effective treatment for cancer or any other disease. Most herbs and supplements may not have been thoroughly tested for interactions with prescribed medicines or cancer therapies.

Overall reduction in processed and red meat, saturated fats, sugar, and alcohol along with an increase in consumption of low-fat foods, fruits and vegetables, and whole grains is associated with better health outcomes for many conditions, including cancer.

What are some potential side effects, cautions, or contraindications?

Some potential effects are nutritional deficiencies that may occur with dietary changes and restrictions, such as deficiencies with calcium, vitamins B_2 and B_{12}, iron, manganese, protein, vitamin D, and zinc.

Where can I learn more?

"Eat a healthy diet, with an emphasis on plant sources," in *ACS Guidelines on Nutrition and Physical Activity for Cancer Prevention,* American Cancer Society, www.cancer.org/Healthy/ EatHealthyGetActive/index

Kushi Institute, www.kushiinstitute.org

"Macrobiotics," American Cancer Society, www.cancer.org/ Treatment/TreatmentsandSideEffects/Complementaryand AlternativeMedicine/DietandNutrition/macrobiotic-diet

Macrobiotics America, www.macroamerica.com

Massage Therapy

What is massage therapy?

Massage therapy is the pressing and/or rubbing of the muscles and soft tissues of the body using the hands and fingers, forearms, elbows, or feet. In Swedish massage, the therapist uses long strokes, kneading, deep circular movements, vibration, and tapping. Other examples are deep tissue massage and trigger point massage, which focuses on relieving muscle knots.

CMT—certified massage therapist

LMT—licensed massage therapist

LMP—licensed massage practitioner

Who practices massage therapy? What certification, licensure, and education options are available?

Approximately 1,500 massage therapy schools and training programs exist in the United States. Massage training programs generally are approved by a state board.

The National Certification Board for Massage Therapy and Bodywork offers certification following a minimum of 500 hours of instruction, mastery of core skills, and passing a standardized exam. As of 2010, 43 states and the District of Columbia had laws regulating massage therapy. In addition to massage therapists, healthcare providers such as chiropractors and physical therapists may have training in massage.

NCTM—nationally certified in therapeutic massage; practitioner has met the credentialing requirements (including passing an exam) of the National Certification Board for Therapeutic Massage and Bodywork for practicing therapeutic massage

NCTMB—nationally certified in therapeutic massage and bodywork; practitioner has met the credentialing requirements (including passing an exam) of the National Certification Board for Therapeutic Massage and Bodywork for practicing therapeutic massage and bodywork

What is the evidence to support the use of massage therapy in cancer care?

Available scientific evidence does not support massage as an effective treatment for cancer or any other disease.

Massage therapy may reduce anxiety, blood pressure, depression, and pain. It also may improve mood and relieve chronic low back pain and neck pain.

What are some potential side effects, cautions, or contraindications?

Massage therapy is generally considered to be safe when performed by a trained therapist. Side effects may include temporary pain or discomfort. Patients with cancer should consult their oncologist before having a massage that involves deep or intense pressure.

Avoid massage in any area of the body with blood clots, fractures, open or healing wounds, skin infections, or known tumor. People with bleeding disorders, those with low blood platelet counts, and those taking blood thinners such as warfarin should avoid deep massage.

Where can I learn more?

"Massage therapy: An introduction," National Center for Complementary and Alternative Medicine, http://nccam.nih.gov/health/massage/massageintroduction.htm

"Massage therapy as an option in supportive care," in *Complementary and Alternative Medicine: Focus on Research and Care*, National Center for Complementary and Alternative Medicine, http://nccam.nih.gov/news/newsletter/2010_september/massage1.htm

Mindfulness Meditation

What is mindfulness meditation?

Meditation refers to a group of techniques, such as concentrative, transcendental, and mindfulness. Meditation focuses attention on one's breathing to develop increased awareness of the present. A person who is meditating uses certain techniques, such as a specific posture, focused attention, and an open attitude toward distractions.

Mindfulness meditation (also called mindfulness-based stress reduction, or MBSR) is a moment-to-moment, present-centered awareness. The goal of MBSR is to guide participants to achieve greater awareness of themselves, their thoughts, and their bodies through class discussion, meditation, and yoga exercises.

Who practices mindfulness meditation? What certification, licensure, and education options are available?

There is no formal credentialing or licensure process for those who practice meditation in its various forms. Many trained practitioners incorporate meditation in their practice. These practitioners may be self-taught or may have taken courses to learn and teach meditation.

What is the evidence to support the use of mindfulness meditation in cancer care?

Available scientific evidence does not support meditation as an effective treatment for cancer or any other disease.

Meditation in its various forms may reduce stress and control emotion, subsequently improving overall health and wellness. Some studies involving meditation are looking into its ability to reduce the frequency and intensity of hot flashes in menopausal women, relieve symptoms of chronic back pain, and improve alertness.

What are some potential side effects, cautions, or contraindications?

Meditation is considered to be safe for healthy people. There have been rare reports that meditation could cause or worsen symptoms in people with some mental or physical health conditions. Individuals should speak with their healthcare providers prior to starting a meditative practice and make their meditation instructor aware of their condition.

People with physical limitations may not be able to participate in certain meditative practices involving physical movement.

Where can I learn more?

"Meditation: An introduction," National Center for Complementary and Alternative Medicine, from http://nccam.nih .gov/health/meditation/overview.htm

Stress Reduction Program, University of Massachusetts Medical School Center for Mindfulness in Medicine, Health Care, and Society, www.umassmed.edu/Content.aspx?id=41254

Also known as European mistletoe, all-heal, bird lime, devil's fuge, golden bough, Iscador®, Eurixor®, Helixor®, Isorel®, Iscucin®, Plenosol®, and ABNOBAviscum®

Mistletoe

What is mistletoe?

Mistletoe is a plant that grows on several species of trees native to Great Britain, Europe, and western Asia. Mistletoe that is found in the United States usually grows on apple, oak, pine, and elm trees. The plant's leaves and twigs are used in herbal remedies; the berries are not used.

Mistletoe preparations vary depending on whether they are extracted with water or alcohol solutions, whether they are fermented or nonfermented, the original species, and the season in which the plant was harvested. In Europe, mistletoe extracts are prescription drugs that are given by injection and used mainly as a treatment for cancer. In the United States, the Food and Drug Administration does not allow injectable mistletoe to be imported, sold, or used except in a research study setting.

What is the evidence to support the use of mistletoe in cancer care?

Available scientific evidence does not support mistletoe as an effective treatment for cancer or any other disease.

Some laboratory experiments suggest that mistletoe extracts may kill cancer cells. Animal studies suggest that mistletoe may be helpful in lessening the side effects of chemotherapy and radiation. Studies to identify the most important components in mistletoe, thought to be the lectins, or proteins, are under way.

What are some potential side effects, cautions, or contraindications?

Purified mistletoe extract is generally considered safe in recommended doses. Possible side effects include temporary redness at the injection site, headaches, fever, and chills. Symptoms of mistletoe toxicity include blurred vision, nausea and vomiting, stomach pain, diarrhea, slow or irregular heartbeat, low blood pressure, confusion, and drowsiness.

Raw, unprocessed mistletoe is poisonous and may lead to seizures, coma, and death. Women who are pregnant or breast-feeding should not use mistletoe.

Where can I learn more?

"Herbs at a glance: European mistletoe," National Center for Complementary and Alternative Medicine, http://nccam.nih .gov/health/mistletoe

"Mistletoe extracts (PDQ®)," National Cancer Institute, www.cancer .gov/cancertopics/pdq/cam/mistletoe/patient

Naturopathy

ND—doctor of naturopathy

What is naturopathy?

Naturopathy is an alternative medical system that combines conventional/traditional medical understanding of human physiology and disease with CAM therapies that are believed to stimulate the body's own natural healing ability.

A naturopathic approach to treating a condition may include nutrition, herbs, acupuncture, bodywork, hydrotherapy, meditation, and counseling.

Who practices naturopathy? What certification, licensure, and education options are available?

Certification is available through the Naturopathic Physicians Licensing Examination Board and the

North American Board of Naturopathic Examiners. Each of the six North American schools is either accredited or a candidate for accreditation by an agency of the U.S. Department of Education.

Licensure requires graduation from a four-year naturopathic medical school and passing a board exam. Fifteen states, the District of Columbia, Puerto Rico, and the U.S. Virgin Islands have licensing laws for naturopathic physicians.

Many trained practitioners incorporate naturopathic methods in their practice. These practitioners may be self-taught or have taken courses on naturopathic methods.

What is the evidence to support naturopathic approaches in cancer care?

Available scientific evidence does not support naturopathy as an effective treatment for cancer or any other disease. Most herbs and supplements may not have been thoroughly tested for interactions with prescribed medicines or cancer therapies.

Antioxidant use, one aspect of naturopathy, is being reviewed in women with breast cancer who are receiving either chemotherapy or radiation therapy. The early and late effects of this use are largely unknown. Investigators are conducting observational studies and clinical trials to reveal the short- and long-term effects of these agents.

What are some potential side effects, cautions, or contraindications?

Limited safety research is available because therapies are often individualized. There are no published reports of serious adverse effects.

Where can I learn more?

American Association of Naturopathic Physicians, www. naturopathic.org/index.asp

"Naturopathic medicine," American Cancer Society, www.cancer. org/Treatment/TreatmentsandSideEffects/Complementary andAlternativeMedicine/MindBodyandSpirit/naturopathic -medicine

"Naturopathy," Healthfinder.gov, U.S. Department of Health and Human Services, www.healthfinder.gov/scripts/SearchContext. asp?topic=1065

Oncology Association of Naturopathic Physicians, www.oncanp.org

Qigong

What is qigong?

Qigong (pronounced "chee kung") is a form of traditional Chinese medicine based on the theory that two opposing yet complementary forces, yin and yang, exist. Qigong is believed to enhance the flow of energy, called "qi," in the body. The process of working toward a smooth flow of qi is called "gong."

Qigong can be a self-trained exercise (internal qigong) or applied by a qigong practitioner (external qigong) bringing together exercise, movement, posture, meditation, and breathing.

Examples of the several types of qigong are tai chi, meditation, yoga, and Reiki.

Who practices qigong? What certification, licensure, and education options are available?

Two certification tracks exist within the National Qigong Association:

- The Qigong Teacher track has four levels ranging from 350 to 1,000 training hours.
- The Clinical Qigong track has two levels, one as a clinical practitioner requiring 500 training hours and 500 didactic hours, and the advanced clinical

therapist requiring 1,500 training hours, 1,000 didactic hours, and minimum of 10 years of clinical experience.

No national standard for Qigong education and credentialing currently exists.

What is the evidence to support the use of qigong in cancer care?

Available scientific evidence does not support qigong as an effective treatment for cancer or any other disease. Also, the current evidence from studies on qigong as supportive cancer care is not conclusive because the number of trials and the sample sizes were too small.

Qigong may promote bone health, cardiopulmonary fitness, balance, and quality of life.

What are some potential side effects, cautions, or contraindications?

Qigong is generally considered safe because of the slow, deliberate movements involved. People who are prone to muscle aches and joint pain may notice these problems if movement or effort is overdone.

A small number of people may become disoriented or anxious and experience some negative feelings. Qigong should not be used by those with a history of mental illness unless under the close supervision of a qualified practitioner.

Where can I learn more?

"A comprehensive review of health benefits of qigong and tai chi," by R. Jahnke, L. Larkey, C. Rogers, J. Etnier, and F. Lin, 2010, *American Journal of Health Promotion, 24*(6), pp. e1–e25. http://dx.doi.org/10.4278/ajhp.081013-LIT-248

"Qigong," American Cancer Society, www.cancer.org/Treatment/TreatmentsandSideEffects/ComplementaryandAlternativeMedicine/MindBodyandSpirit/qigong

Reiki

RP—Reiki practitioner

What is Reiki?

Reiki is an energy therapy based on the belief in a universal energy source that supports the body's own healing nature. Practitioners seek to access this energy, allowing it to flow to the body and facilitate healing.

During Reiki, the practitioner places his or her hands on or just above the patient's body, palms down, using a series of positions. Each position is held until the practitioner feels that the flow of energy has slowed or stopped. A sensation such as heat or tingling in the hand is noted.

Who practices Reiki? What certification, licensure, and education options are available?

Training in traditional Reiki has three levels:

- Each level includes one or more initiations (also known as *attunements* or *empowerments*). Receiving an initiation is believed to activate the ability to access Reiki energy.
- Training for first- and second-degree practice is typically given in 8–12 class hours over two days. Some students seek master-level (third-degree) training. A Reiki master can teach and initiate students. This training may take years.
- No licensing or professional standards currently exist for the practice of Reiki. Certification is available through several groups, such as the American Board of Holistic Practitioners.

What is the evidence to support the use of Reiki in cancer care?

Available scientific evidence does not support Reiki as an effective treatment for cancer or any other disease.

Reiki may improve an individual's overall sense of well-being. Some studies are looking at how Reiki might work, its possible effects on disease progression and anxiety in patients with cancer, and whether it can help reduce nerve pain and cardiovascular risk in people with type 2 diabetes.

What are some potential side effects, cautions, or contraindications?

Reiki is generally considered to be safe and without side effects. Patients may experience a deep state of relaxation during a Reiki session. They might also feel warm, tingly, sleepy, or refreshed.

Where can I learn more?

International Association of Reiki Professionals, www.iarp.org

"Reiki," American Cancer Society, www.cancer.org/Treatment/ TreatmentsandSideEffects/ComplementaryandAlternative Medicine/ManualHealingandPhysicalTouch/reiki

"Reiki: An introduction," National Center for Complementary and Alternative Medicine, http://nccam.nih.gov/health/ reiki/introduction.htm

Yoga

What is yoga?

Yoga is an exercise therapy that involves a program of precise postures, breathing exercises, and meditation aimed at attaining fitness and a healthy lifestyle. More than 100 different types of yoga exist, with the most common type based on hatha yoga.

A typical yoga session starts with the person sitting in an upright position and performing gentle movements, all of which are done very slowly while taking deep breaths from the abdomen. It often ends with the chanting of a mantra to attain a deeper state of relaxation.

Who practices yoga? What certification, licensure, and education options are available?

Many training programs for yoga teachers are available. These programs range from a few days to more than two years and differ depending on the style of yoga. One organization requires at least 200 hours of training, with a specific number of hours in areas including techniques, teaching methodology, anatomy, physiology, and philosophy.

There are no official or well-accepted licensing requirements for yoga teachers in the United States. Many trained practitioners incorporate yoga in their practice. These practitioners may be self-taught or may have taken courses on yoga.

What is the evidence to support the use of yoga in cancer care?

Available scientific evidence does not support yoga as an effective treatment for cancer or any other disease.

Yoga may improve quality of life by relieving some symptoms of chronic diseases. It may also lead to increased relaxation and physical fitness.

What are some potential side effects, cautions, or contraindications?

Some yoga poses that require an individual to become inverted should be avoided in people with spinal disc disease, fragile or atherosclerotic neck arteries, high or low blood pressure, glaucoma, retinal detachment, severe osteoporosis, cervical spondylitis, or any risk for blood clots. A type of yoga called *kapalbhati pranayama* may place excessive pressure on the abdomen, increase blood pressure, and have an adverse outcome in patients with known hypertension.

Where can I learn more?

"Yoga," American Cancer Society, www.cancer.org/Treatment/
TreatmentsandSideEffects/ComplementaryandAlternative
Medicine/MindBodyandSpirit/yoga

Yoga Alliance, http://yogaalliance.org

"Yoga for health: An introduction," National Center for Complementary and Alternative Medicine, http://nccam.nih.gov/
health/yoga/introduction.htm

CHAPTER 3

HERBS, VITAMINS, AND SUPPLEMENTS

T he use of herbs, vitamins, and supplements, also known as *natural products*, is increasing in the United States. In 2007, surveys showed that 18% of American adults reported using these products beyond a multivitamin. Natural products are used for a variety of reasons including health maintenance, health promotion, and prevention and treatment of disease. Most people who use natural products use multiple products for a variety of reasons and do so with other health-related therapies such as exercise, diet, and medications. The concern associated with the use of natural products is that users may believe that *natural* means *safe*. Natural products are not necessarily safe, and what may be safe for one person may not be safe for another. Another misconception is that use of a natural product for one medical condition does not endanger the successful treatment for another. For example, a natural product commonly used for migraine headaches may affect a persons blood-clotting mechanisms, thereby causing a risk for bruising, bleeding, or even hemorrhage. Also, the natural product industry is not regulated in the

"He that takes medicine and neglects diet wastes the skills of the physician."
—Chinese proverb

"To eat is a necessity, but to eat intelligently is an art."
—La Rochefoucauld

United States, and therefore these products may contain inconsistent amounts of the active ingredient or may contain contaminants that could jeopardize user safety. See Understanding Dietary Supplement Labels for more information on dietary supplement regulations and labeling.

> The importance of telling your healthcare provider about any use of natural products cannot be exaggerated—it may save you from a life-threatening reaction.

UNDERSTANDING DIETARY SUPPLEMENT LABELS

Labels on supplements can be very confusing. The Dietary Supplement Health and Education Act was put into effect to expand the definition of dietary supplements and dietary ingredients and required specific information for ingredient and nutrition labeling. The term *dietary supplement* includes not only vitamins and minerals but also herbs, fish oils, enzymes, and combinations of these items. The U.S. Food and Drug Administration says that a dietary supplement includes any product (except tobacco) that

- Is intended to supplement the diet and contains one or more of certain ingredients such as a vitamin, mineral, herb or botanical, or amino acid
- Is any dietary substance used to supplement the diet by increasing total intake
- Is a concentrate, metabolite, constituent, extract, or combination of these
- Is intended for ingestion
- Is labeled as a dietary supplement
- Is not a conventional food.

Product labels can contain a variety of statements and claims, but it is illegal to make claims concerning the use of supplements to diagnose, prevent, treat, or cure specific diseases. For example, a product may not claim to cure or treat cancer. Despite these efforts, labels are still often confusing and contradictory.

Even with all the confusion out there, you can make informed choices. Learning how to read labels when considering supplements can help you better understand and evaluate what may or may not be appropriate for you (of course, consult a healthcare professional before taking any new supplement). The following table shows some abbreviations that often appear on supplement and nutritional labels. (Reprinted from "How to Read Food and Dietary Supplement Labels," by G.M. Decker, 2002, *Clinical Journal of Oncology Nursing, 6*, p. 370.)

Terms Commonly Included on Food and Dietary Supplement Labels

RDA	*Recommended daily allowances* were designed to evaluate groups of people, not individuals. They are based on the needs of healthy people under usual environmental stress but do not address individuals with unique nutritional needs.
RDI	*Reference daily intakes* are for proteins, vitamins, and minerals. These values are based on RDAs.
DRV	*Daily reference values* are measurements of food nutrient components, such as fat and fiber, that do not have established RDAs but do have a relationship with health or wellness.
DRI	*Dietary reference intakes* are revised and updated RDA recommendations. DRIs were established in 1997 and based on 1989 RDAs. They represent a collaborative effort between the United States and Canada.
%DV	*Percent daily value* is a measurement of a particular nutrient in a serving of a food or supplement. It is based on a 2,000-calorie diet.
UTL/UL	*Upper tolerable limit* or *upper limit* represents the maximum amount of a nutrient (i.e., food plus supplemental intake) that can be consumed in a day without adverse effects.

The following examples of supplement labels and the accompanying key can help you to understand the different elements of the label content and what it means to your health. (Reprinted from "How to Read Food and Dietary Supplement Labels," by G.M. Decker, 2002, *Clinical Journal of Oncology Nursing, 6,* p. 372.)

Example 1: Ginkgo Biloba (A)
- Serving size (B): One capsule
- Each capsule contains (D): ginkgo biloba extract (leaf), 0.8% ginkgolide B...40 mg*
* Percent daily value not established (F)

Example 2: Echinacea (A)
- Augustifolia and purpurea
- Each capsule contains (D): Echinacea herbal extract 250 mg* (root and rhizome), (Echinacea purpurea and Echinacea augustifolia) (E); standardized to provide 10 mg phenolic compounds and 37.5 mg polysaccharides; root and rhizome 100 mg* (nonstandardized) (Echinacea augustifolia and Echinacea purpurea) (E)
- Suggested usage (B): Adults: Take one capsule one to four times daily between meals or as directed by physician.
* Percent daily value not established (F)

Example 3: A Vitamin Supplement Label (A)
- Serving size (B): 6 capsules
- Servings per container (C): 10

	Amount per Serving (D)	Percent Daily Value (F, G)
Vitamin A (75% beta-carotene)	20,000 IU	400%
Vitamin C (as ascorbic acid)	500 mg	834%
Vitamin D_3	50 IU	13%
Vitamin E (as dl-alpha-tocopherol acetate E)	200 IU	667%
Thiamin	50 mg	3333%

(Continued on next page)

(Continued)

	Amount per Serving (D)	Percent Daily Value (F, G)
Riboflavin	25 mg	1471%
Niacin (as niacinamide & niacin)	120 mg	600%
Vitamin B$_6$	25 mg	1250%
Folic acid	800 mcg	200%
Calcium (from calcium citrate/ ascorbate complex)	300 mg	30%
Magnesium (from magnesium aspartate/ascorbate complex)	300 mg	75%
Zinc	20 mg	133%
Selenium	200 mcg	286%
Copper	2 mg	100%
PABA (para-aminobenzoic acid)	50 mg	*

* Percent daily value not established (F)

Example 4: Multiple Vitamin/Mineral Trace Element Supplement— Iron Free (A)
* Serving size (B): 6 tablets
* Servings per container (C): 30

	Amount per Serving	Percent Daily Value (F)
Vitamin A (as fish liver oil and 60% [15,000 IU] as natural beta carotene from D. salina)	25,000 IU	500%
Vitamin C (as calcium ascorbate and magnesium/potassium asparate/ascorbate complex)	1,200 mg	200%

(Continued on next page)

(Continued)

	Amount per Serving	Percent Daily Value (F)
Vitamin D₃ (from fish liver oil)	100 IU	25%
Vitamin E (as d-alpha tocopheryl succinate) (E)	400 IU	1333%
Vitamin K₁ (as phytonadione)	60 mcg	75%
Thiamine (as thiamine mononitrate)	100 mg	6667%
Riboflavin	50 mg	2941%
Niacin (as niacinamide and niacin)	200 mg	1000%
Vitamin B₆ (as pyridoxine hydrochloride)	50 mg	2500%
Folic acid	800 mcg	200%
Vitamin B₁₂ (as cyanocobalamin on ion exchange resin)	100 mcg	1667%
Biotin	300 mcg	100%
Pantothenic acid (as d-calcium pantothenate)	400 mg	4000%
Calcium (as calcium citrate and calcium ascorbate)	500 mg	50%
Iodine (from kelp)	150 mcg	100%
Magnesium (as magnesium citrate)	500 mg	125%
Zinc (as zinc aspartate)	20 mg	133%
Selenium (as selenium aspartate)	200 mcg	286%
Copper	2 mg	100%

Other ingredients: modified cellulose gum, methylcellulose, silica, cellulose, vegetable steraine, titanium dioxide, magnesium stearate, gum ghatti, natural tangerine flavor, and canthaxanthin (carotene color)

Key for Examples

(A)   **What is a dietary supplement?** Dietary supplements once were considered to be composed only of essential nutrients such as vitamins, minerals, and proteins. The Dietary Supplement Health and Education Act of 1994 changed the meaning of the term *dietary supplements* to include substances such as herbs, fish oils, enzymes, glandulars, and mixtures of these. Examples 1, 2, 3, and 4 are considered dietary supplements.

(B)   **What is a serving size?** A serving size is stated in amounts familiar to lay consumers (e.g., capsules, tablets, tablespoons, cups). For dietary supplements, a full serving may include several capsules or tablets. Serving sizes of herbs and dietary supplements should not be exceeded; the safety of higher doses has not been established.

(C)   **How many servings are in a container?** Example 1 shows that one capsule is one serving. However, in Example 3, six capsules are one serving; the 60-capsule supply provides only 10 servings, so three bottles would be needed for a one-month supply.

(D)   **What dose is provided in each capsule or tablet?** Example 1 shows that one serving of ginkgo biloba is one capsule. Each capsule contains 0.8% of Ginkgolide B in a 40-milligram dose. Ginkgo's standardization usually is 6% terpene lactones or 0.8% ginkgolide B. In Example 2, the product contains Echinacea augustifolia and Echinacea purpurea. Each Echinacea species has different indications; therefore, consumers should know why a particular product is being used. Example 3 shows that six capsules (a serving) equals 500 mg of vitamin C. Each capsule contains 83.3 mg, or about 142% of the daily value, of vitamin C.

(E)   **How can I tell if a capsule or tablet contains natural or synthetic ingredients?** Example 2 contains Echinacea purpurea and Echinacea augustifolia standardized to provide 10 mg of phenolic compounds. It also contains nonstandardized products. Both are active ingredients in an Echinacea product. They both are "natural" but have different reasons for use. In Example 3, a synthetic Vitamin E is used: dl-alpha tocopherol. Natural vitamin E is d-alpha-tocopherol. Example 4 contains d-alpha-tocopherol, the natural vitamin E. These products are not regulated by the U.S. Food and Drug Administration (FDA), so the percent standardized may not be the same in all products. Knowing what active ingredients are and the names of natural versus synthetic products is the responsibility of consumers.

(F) **What does percent daily value (%DV) mean?** This measurement is helpful because it eliminates the need to understand other measurements, such as milligrams (mg), micrograms (mcg), and international units (IU). %DV provides the amount of a particular nutrient in a serving. FDA has based %DVs on a 2,000-calorie diet. Note. Sugars and protein do not have %DV. Consumers must check ingredient lists to find out what sweeteners have been added. Herbs also have no established %DV (see Examples 1 and 2).

(G) **What does the information at the bottom of a nutrition label mean?** A * used after %DV refers to the information at the bottom of a label: "DVs are based on recommendations for a 2,000-calorie diet." This information must be included on all food labels. Large labels contain even more information, such as "Your daily values may be higher or lower, depending on your calorie needs."

Patients are often confused by information on the Internet and in retail stores, as well as advice from well-meaning friends and family. Reliable resources include your healthcare provider, who can have the products checked for safety and purity by a pharmacy or pharmacist, or your pharmacist, who can check for potential interactions between the natural product and your medications. Other reliable resources include the American Botanical Council (www.abc.herbalgram.org) and consumer newsletters (www.consumerlab.com) where you can check a product's safety and who provide recall information and safety alerts for a particular product. (See the list of reliable resources at the end of this chapter.) Herbal products are rated for safety by the American Herbal Products Association and listed in the *American Herbal Products Association's Botanical Safety Handbook* (edited by M. McGuffin, C. Hobbs, R. Upton, and A. Goldberg, 1997, Boca Raton, FL: CRC Press). Current and updated information is available at www.ahpa.org.

HERBS

What is an herb?

An herb is a plant used for flavor, scent, or medicinal properties. When herbs are used for medicinal or scent properties, any part of the plant may be used, including the leaves, roots, flowers, seeds, resin, root bark, inner bark, berries, and sometimes other portions of the plant. Herbs considered medicinal contain phytochemicals that have an effect on the body. Culinary herbs typically include flowers, leaves, and seeds and are used in small amounts and provide flavor rather than substance to food.

Because herbs, supplements, and vitamins are natural, aren't they safe to use?

Natural does not mean *safe*. *Natural* simply means that something came from nature. Many prescribed and over-the-counter medications also come from nature. There is a risk that they will interact with other herbs or medications, thereby causing a negative or harmful effect.

Can herbs or supplements affect my cancer therapy or other medications?

Herbs are medicines and therefore have the ability to interact with any prescription and over-the-counter medications, other herbs, supplements, and even vitamins.

Is there any research about herbs, supplements, and cancer therapy?

As research continues, we will learn more about the possible risks and potentially dangerous drug interactions. We have learned a lot about herbal products and potential interactions, but much is still unknown. The resources listed in this chapter and throughout the book provide information on the current evidence and research.

My friends are recommending I take some herbs for the side effects of my cancer therapy. Is it okay to take them?

People mean well and want to be helpful, but herbs can affect people differently, and as mentioned earlier, they can interact with drugs you are taking, making them not work properly or even causing other dangerous effects. Refer to the Ten Cardinal Rules of Herb Use for helpful tips.

What are some of the side effects of herbs?

Examples of herbs that can alter blood clotting:

- Alfalfa
- Angelica
- Anise
- Arnica
- Asafoetida
- Bogbean
- Boldo
- Capsicum
- Celery
- Chamomile
- Danshen
- Ephedra
- Fenugreek
- Feverfew
- Garlic
- Ginger
- Ginkgo
- Ginseng
- Goldenseal
- Horse chestnut
- Horseradish
- Licorice
- Meadowsweet
- Onion

- Papain
- Passion flower
- Poplar
- Prickly ash
- Quassia

- Red clover
- Turmeric
- Wild carrot
- Wild lettuce
- Willow

Examples of herbs that can make you feel drowsy or tired:

- Calamus
- Calendula
- California poppy
- Capsicum
- Celery
- Chamomile
- Couch grass
- Elecampane
- Goldenseal
- Gotu kola
- Hops
- Jamaican dogwood
- Kava

- Lemon balm
- Sage
- Sassafras
- Shepherd's purse
- Siberian ginseng
- Skullcap
- St. John's wort
- Stinging nettle
- Valerian
- Wild carrot
- Wild lettuce
- Withania root
- Yerba mansa

Always tell your pharmacist and healthcare providers about all medications, herbs, and natural products that you are taking in order to avoid unwanted reactions.

THE TEN CARDINAL RULES OF HERB USE

Research has shown that patients equate *natural* with *safe*, and some may believe that herbs are organ specific. For example, if antioxidants are used for cardiovascular health, patients may assume that they would not alter cancer therapy. This column is meant to be used as a teaching aid in improving communication between practitioners and patients.

Rule 1: Herbs should not be taken at the same time as any medicine. Taking herbs with prescription medicine or over-the-counter medicine changes the action of one or both.

Rule 2: "When in doubt, do without." If you experience an unpleasant side effect while taking an herb, discontinue immediately. Remember that the so-called "healing crisis" could, in fact, be life threatening.

Rule 3: Learn about herbs before using them. Do not take the advice of people who are not knowledgeable about medicine and herbs.

Rule 4: Accurate diagnosis is essential before using *any* therapy. Many factors should be considered before attempting self-treatment. Do you know or think you know your diagnosis? Guesswork should not be your guide.

Rule 5: Herbal medicines are medicines and should be treated as such. Treat herbal preparations with the same respect you would treat any medicine.

Rule 6: Some herbs are contraindicated in particular health situations. For example, some herbs cause low blood sugar and should not be used by those with hypoglycemia or hyperglycemia (diabetes), and others may alter blood-clotting mechanisms and should be avoided by people taking anticlotting medicines.

Rule 7: Herbs must be taken in specific doses at specific times. For example,
- Vitality and nutrition herbs and herbal formulas are best taken with meals.
- Pain-relief herbs and herbal formulas are best taken between meals.

Rule 8: The effectiveness of an herb depends on a variety of factors, including proper dose, heath status of the person, product quality, and purity.

Rule 9: When purchasing herbs, keep in mind that the best values may be in herb shops or health food stores, but be careful about purity.

Rule 10: Fresh herbs and dried herbs have near-equal advantages when purity is not in question.

Bibliography
Heinerman, J. (1996). *Heinerman's encyclopedia of healing herbs and spices.* New York, NY: Reward Books.

Note. From "The Ten Cardinal Rules of Herb Use," by G.M. Decker, 2006, *Clinical Journal of Oncology Nursing, 10,* p. 279. Copyright 2006 by the Oncology Nursing Society. Reprinted with permission.

COMMONLY USED HERBS AND THEIR POTENTIAL INTERACTIONS

Aloe Vera

What are some common uses?

Aloe has been used as a laxative, anti-inflammatory, and antiviral substance and is often used on the skin to improve healing.

Does it have any potential interactions?

Potential interactions include licorice, drugs used to treat diabetes, insulin, and digoxin.

Aloe vera should not be used by patients with inflammatory bowel disease, appendicitis, abdominal pain, irregular heartbeats, neuropathy, or swelling of extremities.

What are the known side effects?

Potential side effects include abdominal cramping, dehydration, delayed healing, diarrhea, hepatitis, low blood sugar, low potassium levels, irregular heartbeat, rash, thyroid problems, and uterine spasms. With long-term use, it can cause bone loss.

Bilberry

What are some common uses?

Bilberry has been used as an astringent, as an antioxidant, and to protect or improve circulation.

Does it have any potential interactions?

Use caution; you should not use bilberry if you are taking anticoagulants, including low-molecular-weight heparin and aspirin.

What are the known side effects?

Potential side effects include bleeding (increased risk if taken with blood thinners), heartburn, low blood sugar, and increased blood pressure.

Chamomile

What are some common uses?

Chamomile has been used for its mild sedative effect, to lower blood sugar, for its estrogen effects, and as an antiseptic.

Does it have any potential interactions?

Potential interactions include blood thinners, prescription and over-the-counter nonsteroidal anti-inflammatory drugs (NSAIDs), aspirin (increased bleeding), acetaminophen, dextromethorphan/pseudoephedrine (cough medicines), sedatives, herbs that cause sedation, antidepressants, capsaicin, dong quai, primrose oil, fenugreek, feverfew, fish oil, garlic, ginger, ginkgo biloba, ginseng, horse chestnut, licorice, and St. John's wort.

What are the known side effects?

With topical use, potential side effects include burning of the face, eyes, and mucous membranes. With systemic (oral) use, possible side effects include bleeding, bruising, confusion, drowsiness, and severe allergic reaction (anaphylaxis).

Cinnamon

What are some common uses?

Cinnamon has been used as an antifungal, antiseptic, analgesic, and antiviral and to lower blood sugar and blood pressure.

Does it have any potential interactions?

To date there are no known or potential interactions with drugs and other herbs.

What are the known side effects?

Potential side effects include flushing, increased heart rate, mouth sores, sore tongue, loss of appetite, dermatitis, shortness of breath, and increased stomach and intestinal action (motility). People with current or past stomach ulcers should use caution with or avoid use of cinnamon. There is a report of a squamous cell cancer of the tongue with repeated and prolonged use of cinnamon-flavored gum.

Echinacea

What are some common uses?

Echinacea has been used as an antiviral, to stimulate the immune system, and to treat psoriasis.

Does it have any potential interactions?

Avoid use with immune modulators (for example, cyclosporine, protease inhibitors, corticosteroids, methotrexate, and any drug that suppresses the immune system). Avoid use with amiodarone, camptothecins, epidermal growth factor receptor tyrosine kinase inhibitors (EGFR-TKIs), epipodophyllotoxins, ketoconazole, methotrexate, taxanes, and vinca alkaloids. Also avoid if you have an autoimmune disorder or are allergic to daisy and chrysanthemum (because of an increased risk of hypersensitivity reaction). Echinacea may alter drugs used to suppress the immune system and birth control pills

What are the known side effects?

Potential side effects include liver toxicity, acute asthma attack, severe allergic reactions; may increase liver enzyme tests, lymphocyte counts, and sedimentation rate. People with altered lymphocytes, immunoglobulin G (or IgG), and sedimentation rate should avoid use of echinacea.

Garlic

What are some common uses?

Garlic has been used as an antioxidant and to lower cholesterol level.

Does it have any potential interactions?

Avoid use with dacarbazine (also known as DTIC). Also avoid use with other chemotherapy because safety data remain inconclusive as of the printing of this book. Avoid use before or immediately after surgery because of its effect on the blood's ability to clot. It has potential interactions with anticoagulants and any drug, herb, or supplement that has anticoagulant properties (such as aspirin, NSAIDs, vitamin E [greater than 400 IU]).

What are the known side effects?

Potential side effects include bad breath, changed taste, low blood sugar, lower cholesterol levels, and increased prothrombin time, international normalized ratio (known as INR), and immunoglobulin E (or IgE).

Ginkgo Biloba

What are some common uses?

Ginkgo biloba has been used to help improve memory, as an antioxidant, to improve circulation, and to decrease pain.

Does it have any potential interactions?

Potential interactions include many anticancer drugs, such as camptothecin (topotecan, irinotecan), cyclophosphamide

(Cytoxan®), EGFR-TKIs, epipodophyllotoxins (etoposide, teniposide), taxanes (Taxol®, Taxotere®), vinca alkaloids (vincristine, vinblastine), alkylating agents, antitumor antibiotics, and platinum analogs.

Other interactions include anticoagulants and any drug, herb, or vitamin with anticoagulant properties (for example, NSAIDs, aspirin, vitamin E [greater than 400 IU], garlic, and ginseng).

What are the known side effects?

Potential side effects include reports of subarachnoid hemorrhage (bleeding in the brain), altered blood clotting, anxiety, restlessness, stomach and intestinal symptoms, skin reactions, and increased insulin levels.

Ginseng

What are some common uses?

Ginseng has been used for increasing physical endurance and stamina and to help alleviate stress and fatigue.

Does it have any potential interactions?

Potential interactions exist with acetaminophen, some anesthetics, anticoagulants, antidepressants, antihistamines and antihistamine/decongestant combinations, aspirin, barbiturates, benzodiazepines, calendula, cannabinoids, capsicum, cardiac medications, chamomile, dextromethorphan, digoxin, diphenhydramine, drugs or herbs that alter blood clotting, fenugreek, gabapentin (Neurontin®), goldenseal, gotu kola, heparins, hydrocodone, ibritumomab tiuxetan (Zevalin®), kava, lemon balm, melatonin, methadone, muscle relaxants, NSAIDs, oxycodone, pseudoephedrine, selective serotonin reuptake inhibitors, thyroid medications, and valerian.

Ginseng should be used with caution or avoided in people with fever, hypertension, autoimmune disorders, breast cancer, coronary artery disease, endometriosis, endometrial cancer, hormone-sensitive conditions, ovarian cancer, history of heart attack, rheumatic heart disease, or psychiatric disorders and people taking antidepressants.

Avoid use with camptothecins, cyclophosphamide, EGFR-TKIs, epipodophyllotoxins, taxanes, and vinca alkaloids. Do not take ginseng if you have estrogen receptor–positive breast or endometrial cancer.

What are the known side effects?

Potential side effects include aggressive behavior, irritability, anxiety, nervousness, palpitations, rapid heart rate, estrogen-like effects and other hormone influence, breast tenderness, headache, hypoglycemia, and hypertension.

Kava
What are some common uses?

Kava has been used for a sedative effect, to relax the skeletal muscles, and as an anti-inflammatory.

Does it have any potential interactions?

Potential interactions include drugs used to treat Parkinson disease, psychiatric medications, barbiturates, and any drug the depresses the central nervous system. Other interactions include benzodiazepines, dopamine antagonists, and ethanol (alcohol). Kava increases the effect of barbiturates and intensifies psychoactive agents.

Avoid use with camptothecins, cyclophosphamide, EGFR-TKIs, epipodophyllotoxins, taxanes, and vinca alkaloids and in combination with any chemotherapy that is potentially toxic to the liver. Do not take kava if you have existing liver disease, evidence of liver damage, or herb-induced liver toxicity.

What are the known side effects?

Potential side effects include drowsiness, blurred vision, nausea, vomiting, loss of appetite, shortness of breath, and allergic reactions; decreased platelets, lymphocytes, bilirubin, protein, and albumin; and increased red blood cell volume and liver function tests.

Milk Thistle
What are some common uses?
Milk thistle has been used to protect the liver, as treatment for cirrhosis of the liver caused by alcohol or virus, and as an anti-inflammatory and antioxidant.

Does it have any potential interactions?
Potential interactions include warfarin and other drugs that alter blood clotting; combination products that contain acetaminophen, dextromethorphan, and pseudoephedrine; and estrogen and progestin. Milk thistle may decrease levels of irinotecan, lorazepam, lovastatin, morphine, and meprobamate.

What are the known side effects?
Potential side effects include headache, nausea, vomiting, diarrhea, loss of appetite, abdominal bloating, abdominal pain, menstrual changes, allergic reactions, erectile dysfunction, pruritus (itching of the skin), and joint pain. It also may decrease liver function tests and blood glucose levels.

St. John's Wort
What are some common uses?
St. John's wort has been used for anxiety, dermatitis, mild to moderate depression, insomnia, migraines, and seasonal affective disorder.

Does it have any potential interactions?
Use with caution or avoid St. John's wort if you have dementia, bipolar disorder, or diabetes or are

psychotic or suicidal. Also avoid use with anesthesia, antidepressants (monoamine oxidase inhibitors and selective serotonin reuptake inhibitors), antifungals, any concurrent chemotherapy (examples include but are not limited to cyclosporine, etoposide, and irinotecan), digoxin, immunosuppressants, indinavir and other protease inhibitors, oral contraceptives, theophylline, verapamil, warfarin and other anticoagulants, and many other drugs. It should not be used with other medications, herbs, or supplements.

Also avoid use if you have sensitivity to *Hypericum perforatum* (specific plant), with tyramine-containing foods (such as cheese, meat, fish, and yeast beans), and prior to surgery.

What are the known side effects?

Potential side effects include abdominal pain, abnormal dreams, agitation, alopecia, anorexia, anxiety, constipation, sweating, diarrhea, dizziness, dry mouth, indigestion, fatigue, swelling, headache, high blood pressure, insomnia, irritability, rapid heart rate, muscle cramps, nausea, numbness, itching, restlessness, and weakness. It has additive effects with antidepressants including increased sensitivity to ultraviolet light and sunlight, rashes, gastrointestinal symptoms (nausea), dizziness, confusion, sedation, fatigue, dry mouth, restlessness, anxiety, headache, and alterations in clotting.

A Few Final Thoughts

Always tell your pharmacist and healthcare providers about all medications, herbs, and natural products that you are taking to avoid an unwanted reaction. The herbs that you are interested in using may be effective for a symptom you are experiencing, but they may not be safe for you to take at this time. Always consider your current medications and therapies. As noted by Dr. David M. Eisenberg of Beth Israel Deaconess Medical Center: "Safety trumps efficacy."

You can help in the safe use of herbs and natural products. The U.S. Food and Drug Administration's MedWatch program provides current safety information on drugs, dietary supplements, devices, and cosmetics. E-mails and postings on the MedWatch Web site contain information about adverse events. You can report any reaction you experience by accessing the MedWatch Online Voluntary Reporting Form at www.accessdata.fda .gov/scripts/medwatch/ medwatch-online.htm or by calling 800-FDA-1088 (800-332-1088). A toll-free information line is also available for consumers at 888-INFO-FDA (888-463-6332).

Natural products that can interact with . . .

- **Alcoholic beverages** and cause impairment, sleepiness, or toxicity: chamomile, kava, lavender, St. John's wort, lemon balm
- **Antacids and medications that decrease stomach acid** and interfere in the action of the medication or cause sedation: acidophilus, capsicum, ginger, lavender, peppermint
- **Anticoagulants and medications that are used to control blood clotting** and alter the action of the medication, cause stomach irritation, and increase risk of bleeding: acidophilus, bilberry, chamomile, fish oil, ginkgo, ginseng, garlic
- **Antidiabetic medications** and increase or decrease their effect: aloe, bilberry, flax, garlic, ginseng
- **Anticancer drugs** and interfere with the action of the drug or increase the drug's toxicity: acidophilus, ginseng, milk thistle, soy, St. John's wort
- **NSAIDs** and increase or decrease the action of the drug or increase risk for bleeding: bilberry, garlic, ginkgo, ginseng, St. John's wort

VITAMINS

What is a vitamin?

Vitamins are organic substances needed in very small amounts for normal growth and activity in the body.

Do I need to take vitamins?

Vitamins are supplements and therefore are meant to supplement your diet. Not everyone needs to take vitamins. People who do not get enough nutrients through the foods they eat may need to supplement with vitamins. Some people should not take vitamin supplements because of potential interactions with their cancer therapy or medications they may be taking for other conditions. Seek the help of a healthcare professional (not a diet program or well-meaning friends and neighbors). One recommendation is to begin with a high-quality multivitamin. Do not take any supplement that contains food coloring or preservatives. This information will be on the label, usually listed under "other ingredients." There is a pocket-size publication available that can assist you: *Food Additives: A Shopper's Guide to What's Safe and What's Not* (Revised Edition), 2007, by Christine Hoza Farlow, D.C., published by and available from KISS For Health Publishing, Escondido, CA (www.healthyeatingadvisor. com). You can also order it through your local bookstore or online retailers.

Which vitamins are fat soluble and water soluble, and why does it matter if they are fat or water soluble?

Vitamins A, D, E, and K are fat soluble. Fat-soluble vitamins are soluble (able to be dissolved) in lipids (fats).

These vitamins, especially vitamins A and E, are then stored in body tissues. Once they have been stored in tissues, they tend to remain there. This means that if a person takes in too much of a fat-soluble vitamin, over time the individual can have too much of that vitamin present in the body, a condition called *hypervitaminosis* (too much vitamin in the body). The excess is stored in the liver as fatty tissue. People can also be deficient in the fat-soluble vitamins if their fat intake is too low or if their fat absorption is compromised.

The B vitamins and vitamin C are water soluble. This means they are dissolved in water and transported through the body. Water-soluble vitamins are not stored in the body, and therefore hypervitaminosis is not an issue. If a person consumes too much of a water-soluble vitamin, the excess is excreted in the urine. Regular intake, through foods and possibly supplements, is needed to meet the body's needs.

What do I need to know about the different vitamins?

Vitamin A (retinol)

Carotenes are antioxidants that are slowly changed by the body to vitamin A (retinol). Food sources include liver, dairy products, and fish. Food sources of vitamin A precursor (also known as provitamin A) beta-carotene include vegetables such as carrots, sweet potatoes, spinach, and other green leafy vegetables, and fruit such as cantaloupes and apricots.

Too much carotene in the diet can temporarily yellow the skin. Too little may lead to vitamin A deficiency. Deficiency of vitamin A is considered a serious health problem; it can cause joint pain or diarrhea and may lead to night blindness.

Some prescribed medications can interfere with absorption. Vitamin E, vitamin C, thyroid hormones, and zinc decrease the functions of vitamin A.

Adults need 700–1,000 mcg per day. Supplements of vitamin A should be taken only under the supervision of a healthcare professional. High doses can be toxic and are believed to increase the risk for lung cancer in those who smoke. Research has shown that beta-carotene is not likely to provide cancer prevention and may cause harm to some groups.

Vitamin B₁ (thiamin)

Vitamin B_1 works in the body as a coenzyme needed for energy production, metabolism, and kidney cell function. Food sources include soybeans, brown rice, sunflower seeds, peanuts, most whole grains, fruit, legumes, seafood, and meat products.

Adults need 0.9–1.5 mg per day. Deficiency is rare except in alcoholics and people with chronic illness. Symptoms of deficiency include fatigue, depression, and constipation, and deficiency is associated with diseases of the heart and nervous system. Alcohol, tannins (tea, coffee), and uncooked freshwater fish can destroy thiamin. Long-term use of some diuretics may cause a deficiency.

Vitamin B₂ (riboflavin)

Vitamin B_2 plays a role in energy production and has antioxidant properties. Food sources include organ meats, almonds, mushrooms, whole grains, soybeans, and green leafy vegetables.

Adults need 1.2–1.7 mg per day; the need decreases with age. Deficiency is rare but does occur in the elderly. Deficiency can cause cracks at the corner of the mouth or lips, inflammation of the lining of the mouth and skin, itching of the eyes, mouth, and tongue, and anemia. Deficiency should be medically supervised.

Riboflavin may strengthen vitamin E antioxidant action. It can cause false highs and lows in some blood tests and stool tests for invisible blood. Some cholesterol-lowering drugs, antidepressants, birth control pills, and laxatives can decrease riboflavin absorption. Supplements can cause bright yellow discoloration of urine.

Vitamin B_3 (niacin)

Vitamin B_3 is needed for body metabolism. Tryptophan is converted to niacin by the body. Food sources include organ meats, eggs, fish, peanuts, legumes, whole grains (except corn), milk, and avocados.

Adults need 13–19 mg per day; the need decreases with age. Severe deficiency causes dermatitis, dementia, and diarrhea.

Vitamin B_3 is contraindicated in people with liver disease, high liver enzymes, gout, and peptic ulcers. It should be used with caution as a supplement in patients with diabetes and cancer.

Potential interactions include some blood pressure, heart, diabetes, and anticholesterol medications; red yeast rice; and ethanol-containing food and beverages (typically beer and liquors, but some foods can create small amounts of ethanol through fermentation). Side effects of supplementation include flushing, nausea, vomiting, diarrhea, headaches, and dizziness. Time-released supplements lower the risk of flushing but can cause liver toxicity and weaken glucose tolerance.

Vitamin B₆ (pyridoxine)

Vitamin B$_6$ works with enzymes in the formation of body proteins and other processes needed by the body. Food sources include meat, poultry, fish, eggs, white potatoes, starchy vegetables, non-citrus fruits, fortified cereals, fortified soy-based meat substitutes, whole grains, legumes, bananas, seeds, nuts, brussels sprouts, and cauliflower.

Adults need 1.6–2 mg per day. Deficiency leads to cracking of the lips, inflammation of the tongue and mouth, anemia, irritability, altered glucose tolerance, confusion, and depression. Chronic intake of alcohol can cause deficiency. Less obvious symptoms of deficiency can be seen with malabsorption, cancer, heart failure, and cirrhosis and in the elderly.

High doses may cause nausea, vomiting, abdominal pain, loss of appetite, and sensitivity to light. Potential interactions include theophylline and some medications used to treat high blood pressure and Parkinson disease.

Vitamin B₁₂ (cobalamin)

Vitamin B$_{12}$ is stored in the liver, kidneys, and other body tissues and works with folate for important body processes. It is needed in the genetic material of all cells. Food sources include liver, kidney, eggs, fish, cheese, and meat.

Adults need 1.8–2.4 mcg per day. Strict vegetarian diets can result in deficiency. Deficiency can lead to anemia, tingling and numbness of extremities, abnormalities of standing (balance) and walking, constipation alternating with diarrhea, abdominal pain, inflammation of the tongue, loss of appetite, and weight loss.

Allergic reactions have been reported, including itching, rash, and hives. Potential interactions include some cholesterol-lowering medications and metformin. Acid-blocking drugs decrease the absorption of B_{12} from food but not from supplements.

Folate (folic acid)

Folic acid is a B vitamin. It functions with vitamin B_{12}. Food sources include dark green leafy vegetables, oranges, lentils, pinto beans, garbanzo beans, asparagus, broccoli, cauliflower, liver, and brewer's yeast.

Adults need 200–400 mcg per day. Deficiency is caused by alcoholism, malabsorption syndromes, and small intestine surgeries. Dialysis and some chronic skin conditions can cause an increased need for folate. Supplementation with doses greater than 400 mcg should be medically supervised.

Potential interactions include antiseizure drugs that have lithium activity, NSAIDs, methotrexate, hormone replacement therapy, and birth control pills. Toxicities are seen with doses greater than 1,000 mcg and may worsen neurologic damage seen with B_{12} deficiency or can increase seizure activity in people with epilepsy.

Vitamin C (ascorbic acid, ascorbate)

Vitamin C is an antioxidant, aids in wound healing and iron absorption, increases the level of good cholesterol, and is essential for healthy gums, teeth, bones, and blood vessels. Food sources include oranges, lemons, grapefruit, and their juices and cantaloupe, honeydew, watermelon, kiwi, papaya, strawberries, asparagus, broccoli, cauliflower, mustard greens, peppers, potatoes, and tomatoes.

Should I take a multivitamin every day?
You should discuss this with your healthcare providers to be sure there are no potential interactions given your health and medication profile.

Adults need 60–90 mg per day. Deficiency can lead to bruising, petechiae (small red or purple spots), mild anemia, slow wound healing, depression, hair loss, and edema (swelling).

Potential interactions include antacids that contain aluminum, cyclosporine, and cholesterol-lowering drugs. It may alter cisplatin, doxorubicin, and paclitaxel and increases the uptake of non-heme iron. It may regenerate vitamin E, causes a false increase in bilirubin and creatine in urine and blood, and can cause false-positives in stool tests for blood. It is contraindicated in people with preexisting kidney disease, history of kidney stones, altered kidney function, hemochromatosis, thalassemia, sickle-cell anemia, and G6PD deficiency. With doses greater than 2–3 grams per day, nausea, vomiting, abdominal cramping, and gas may occur

To date, clinical trials looking at the effect of vitamin C in cancer prevention have not shown benefit.

Vitamin D (cholecalciferol)

Vitamin D is synthesized in the skin and is best known for stimulating calcium absorption. It is believed to have anti–bone loss effects and immune, cell growth and death, anticancer, antioxidant, anti-inflammatory, and mood action. Sunlight is a source of vitamin D. Few food sources exist except for fatty fish, fish liver oils, and eggs from hens fed vitamin D. Most vitamin D is found in fortified foods such as milk and cereals.

Adult requirements are based on blood tests. Deficiency can lead to osteomalacia (soft bones) in adults and bone deformity (rickets) in children. People at risk for deficiency include the elderly, those with limited sun exposure, people with dark skin, those with malabsorption (such as people with celiac disease, Crohn disease, or chronic liver disease), those who have had gastric surgeries, and those who are obese.

Potential interactions include some cholesterol-lowering drugs, phenobarbital, and phenytoin (Dilantin®), which lower vitamin D levels. Thiazide diuretics and vitamin D may cause hypercalcemia.

There is increasing interest and research in the role that vitamin D may play in cancer care. An increasing number of studies are suggesting that higher vitamin D concentrations in the blood are associated with lower rates of different cancer types. It is not currently known whether changing an individual's vitamin D concentration over time is beneficial. The Vitamin D and Omega 3 Trial (VITAL) is ongoing research looking at the potential benefits of fish oil supplementation on overall cancer risk (see www.ClinicalTrials.gov, ClinicalTrials.gov identifier NCT01169259).

Vitamin E (tocopherol)

Vitamin E is a family of eight related components. It is important in the development of the central nervous system and is an antioxidant and retina protectant. It is found in food but in small amounts. Food sources include green leafy vegetables, some green, brown, and blue-green algae, unrefined vegetable oils, nuts, grains, and fortified cereal. Vitamin E is destroyed by heat processing.

Adults may need 15 1,000 IUs per day. Deficiencies are not common but occur in people with fat malabsorption, pancreatic enzyme deficiency, cystic fibrosis, and short bowel syndrome. Symptoms of deficiency include tingling or loss of sensation in extremities, loss of specific reflexes and sense of balance and coordination, muscle weakness, and specific changes in eyesight.

Potential interactions include some cholesterol-lowering drugs, sucralfate (Carafate®), antiseizure drugs, anticoagulants, some cancer chemotherapy, verapamil, ginseng, ginkgo, and garlic, which will enhance anticlotting. Dietary fiber can decrease the antioxidant effects. Supplements should contain mixed tocopherols.

Toxicities can be seen with doses higher than 1,200 mg per day and include muscle fatigue, breast tenderness, gastrointestinal upset, and thyroid problems. No benefit of vitamin E on the prevention of breast, lung, or colon cancer has been shown.

Vitamin K (menadione)

Vitamin K is needed for normal blood clotting. K_1 is the primary dietary source. Food sources include green leafy vegetables, vegetable oils, chicken, egg yolk, butter, cow liver, some cheeses, and some fermented soybean products.

Deficiency is rare but can be caused by inadequate intake or malabsorption. Symptoms include bruising, nosebleeds, blood in the urine, and heavy menstruation.

Potential interactions include anticlotting medications and herbs, some antibiotics, warfarin, Dilantin, mineral oil, and some cholesterol-lowering medications. Vitamins A and E interfere with vitamin K.

Toxicity is seen with K_3; it is not a nutritional supplement. Supplements should be taken *only* with medical supervision.

SUPPLEMENTS

Calcium

An essential mineral involved in several body processes, calcium is needed to prevent and treat osteoporosis. Food sources include milk products, collard greens, Chinese cabbage, mustard greens, broccoli, bok choy, tofu, and sardines with bones. It is poorly absorbed from food with oxalic acid: spinach, sweet potatoes, rhubarb, beans, unleavened bread, seeds, nuts, and grains.

Adults need 800–1,500 mg per day. Deficiency causes osteoporosis. Supplement absorption varies with the different types: carbonate, citrate, phosphate, lactate, or gluconate. It is best absorbed in doses of 500 mg or less with up to 250 mg magnesium. People with low stomach acid (those who take acid-blocking drugs or in achlorhydria) best absorb carbonate. Caution is necessary if taking supplements without food, as this increases the risk for kidney stones. Calcium supplementation is contraindicated in those with history of calcium-containing kidney stones. Carbonate may cause bloating, constipation, and gas.

Potential interactions include decreased absorption of bisphosphonates, acid-reducing medications, levothyroxine, quinolone, and tetracycline if taken concurrently with calcium. Iron, fluoride, magnesium, phosphorus, and zinc decrease calcium absorption.

Coenzyme Q10 (ubiquinone)

Coenzyme Q10, or CoQ10, is involved in energy production in cells. Many benefits have been proposed, including an effect on heart and blood vessels. It does not help with weight loss as has been claimed. Food sources include all foods; it is present in every plant and animal. Piperine (in black pepper) may increase CoQ10 levels in the blood.

No established daily recommendation exists for adults. Deficiency states can occur in those with inflammation of the gums (gingivitis). The supplement is best taken with foods that contain fat. Absorption is approximately 40% of the dose taken.

Potential interactions include warfarin, cholesterol-lowering drugs, antidiabetic medications, and beta-blockers (e.g., propranolol).

Fish oils, marine oils; omega-3s

EPA and DHA, or fish oil, has a positive effect on the cardiovascular system, anti-inflammation, and brain function. Food sources include fish (especially coldwater fish).

No dietary requirement has been set, and deficiency states have not been established. Side effects include nausea, diarrhea, and bad breath. Some supplements are enteric coated to avoid bad breath.

Caution is necessary for people on anticlotting drugs and herbs, as fish oils may enhance these effects, causing bruising, nosebleeds, bleeding gums, and blood in the urine and stool. Toxicity can result if fish oil is taken with vitamins A and D.

Currently, research suggests that EPA and DHA may protect against colorectal cancer in high-risk populations. The Vitamin D and Omega-3 Trial (VITAL) is ongoing research looking at the potential benefits of fish oil supplementation on overall cancer risk.

Iron

Iron is an essential trace element for humans. Its major action is to prevent or treat iron-deficiency anemia. Food sources include green vegetables, legumes, and meat. Iron in bread and cereal is not absorbed well.

Adults need 10–15 mg per day. Deficiency without anemia can cause muscle weakness and exercise fatigue. Low levels are associated with restless legs syndrome.

Potential interactions include acid-blocking medications, levodopa, levothyroxine, tetracycline and quinolone antibiotics, vitamin C, calcium, magnesium, and zinc. Iron supplementation is contraindicated in people with hemochromatosis and those with anemias other than iron-deficiency anemia. It can be toxic to children.

Side effects include nausea, vomiting, bloating, black stool, diarrhea, constipation, and loss of appetite. Liquid preparations will cause staining of teeth. Medical supervision is needed for treatment of iron-deficiency anemia.

Magnesium

Magnesium is an essential mineral absorbed from the small intestine and colon. It produces cellular energy, protein synthesis, and muscle contraction. It also acts as a laxative and antacid. Food sources include tofu, nuts, green vegetables, and unpolished grains. Diets high in refined foods, meat, and dairy interfere with consuming adequate amounts of magnesium.

Adults need 280–350 mg daily. The elderly are at increased risk for deficiency because of a decreased ability to absorb the mineral. Other risk factors for deficiency include alcohol consumption, surgery, diuretic use, liver or kidney disease, or use of birth control pills. Symptoms of deficiency include anorexia, nausea, vomiting, diarrhea, muscle spasms and cramping, fatigue, mental confusion, irritability, tremors, loss of coordination, tingling and numbness in extremities, irregular heartbeat, and vasospasm (spasm of blood vessels). Deficiency can cause hypokalemia (low potassium).

Potential interactions include diuretics, cisplatin, amphotericin, intravenous pentamidine, and cyclosporine. Magnesium decreases absorption of bisphosphonates, quinolones, tetracycline, iron, manganese, and foods rich in oxalic acid (spinach, sweet potatoes, rhubarb, beans) or phytic acid (unleavened bread, raw beans, seeds, nuts, grains).

Magnesium supplementation is contraindicated in people with renal failure, myasthenia gravis, and specific cardiac conditions (atrioventricular block). Supplements are easily absorbed when taken orally. Abdominal cramping and nausea occur with daily doses higher than 350 mg.

Selenium

Selenium is considered an essential trace element (required only in small amounts) and an antioxidant. The amount in food is dependent on the amount in the soil, which varies; therefore, deficiencies and toxicities (with high amounts) are possible.

Adults need 70–200 mcg per day. Food sources include wheat germ, Brazil nuts, oats, whole wheat bread, bran, barley, orange juice, turnips, garlic, and brown rice. Deficiency occurs with specific conditions (for example, some heart conditions, Kashin-Beck disease).

Toxicity is called *selenosis.* Symptoms include depression, nervousness, emotional instability, nausea, vomiting, and garlic odor of breath and sweat. Severe toxicity can cause loss of hair and fingernails.

Selenium has no known interactions with drugs. Cancer chemotherapy may increase a person's need for selenium. Higher doses require medical supervision. Current research has shown that selenium has not reduced the incidence of skin cancer. Research also has suggested a possibility of increased risk for bladder cancer, breast cancer, melanoma, head and neck cancer, lymphoma, and leukemia with use of selenium supplements.

Zinc

Considered an essential trace element, zinc is used for protein metabolism and energy production. Food sources include shellfish (especially oysters), fish, red meats, whole grains, legumes, nuts, and seeds.

Adults need 8–15 mg per day. Deficiency is not common but does occur with alcoholism, malabsorption, and anorexia nervosa. Night blindness has been associated with deficiency states.

Potential interactions include bisphosphonates, quinolone antibiotics and tetracycline, calcium, copper, iron, phosphate salts, and coffee and caffeine. Foods containing oxalic acid (spinach, sweet potatoes, rhubarb, beans) decrease absorption of zinc. Zinc can interfere with cisplatin.

Toxicity is rare. Doses higher than 30 mg per day can cause nausea, vomiting, gastrointestinal discomfort, metallic taste, headache, and drowsiness. Long-term use of zinc supplements can lead to copper deficiency.

RESOURCES

American Botanical Council, www.abc.herbalgram.org
American Herbal Products Association, www.ahpa.org
Natural Medicines Comprehensive Database, www.naturaldatabase
.com
Natural Standard database, www.naturalstandard.com
Richters Herbs, www.herbs.com

CHAPTER 4

SYMPTOM MANAGEMENT WITH COMPLEMENTARY AND ALTERNATIVE MEDICINE

Symptoms of cancer may begin before diagnosis and may extend long after cancer treatment is over. Rarely are symptoms absent. More often, people have a spectrum of symptoms, some more distressing, some less distressing, some that come and go, and some that are long term and never resolve. Although new options for symptom relief are available, many physical, emotional, spiritual, and psychological long-term consequences remain. The impact of symptoms on everyday life is untold.

Symptom clusters are two or more symptoms that are sometimes seen together. These symptoms may have different causes and different time lengths. Some examples are

• Cough, breathlessness, and fatigue
• Dyspnea (shortness of breath), anxiety, and fatigue
• Fatigue, pain, anxiety, and depression
• Nausea, anorexia, and dehydration
• Pain and depression
• Pain, fatigue, and sleep disturbances.

Surveys show that CAM use is widespread in cancer symptom management. Use of a CAM therapy, however, does not mean that it is safe and effective. Some CAM therapies, though, can be safely used and have proven efficacy. It is not uncommon for patients to use both conventional and CAM approaches to relieve symptoms and side effects. In this guide, the symptoms and side effects will be discussed under the umbrella of symptom management.

Cutaneous complications include skin and nail bed changes, skin reactions to targeted therapies, hand-foot syndrome (also known as palmar-plantar erythrodysesthesia), rash with epidermal growth factor receptor inhibitors, and radiation dermatitis.

Many magazines, Web sites, and professional journals focus on the symptoms for which more interest or more information exists. These symptoms are listed below in categories:

- "Up-and-coming" symptoms gaining more attention: cutaneous complications (skin and nail), infertility, neuralgia (nerve pain), sexuality and sexual health
- "Popular" symptoms: fatigue, mucositis (mouth sores), nausea and vomiting
- Distressing symptoms without a wide range of effective conventional or CAM interventions: anorexia-cachexia syndrome (loss of appetite/wasting of body tissue), neuropathies (nerve pain in the hands and/or feet), xerostomia (dry mouth).

Before using any CAM therapy for any symptom or condition, you must be sure of the cause of that symptom or condition. An accurate diagnosis is essential for successful treatment. See your healthcare provider and discuss your symptom or condition and the CAM therapy you are considering. For example, fatigue can be caused by anemia, a sleep disorder, nutritional deficits, and depression. An accurate diagnosis is fundamental to safe and appropriate treatment. And remember, all treatments and therapies have potential side effects. Even though a therapy may have the potential to be effective for your symptom, it may cause a side effect that could be a problem for you (thus making it not safe). Safety always comes first. If there is any doubt, do without.

This next section addresses many symptoms with the focus on the following questions: Which CAM therapies are available to treat this condition? Are any CAM therapies being studied for this condition? The last section of this chapter provides more information on CAM use in pediatric, adolescent, and geriatric populations.

ANOREXIA-CACHEXIA SYNDROME (LOSS OF APPETITE/WASTING OF BODY TISSUE)

What is anorexia-cachexia syndrome?

Anorexia is the loss of appetite or desire to eat. It may be a result of the cancer itself or its treatment. *Cachexia* is a progressive wasting syndrome, and anorexia can contribute to the course of cachexia. Anorexia-cachexia syndrome is a loss of appetite and weight, tissue wasting, and decreases in muscle mass and adipose tissue.

Many other symptoms negatively contribute to this syndrome, such as mucositis (mouth sores), taste alterations, xerostomia (dry mouth), pain, dyspnea (shortness of breath), and depression. Nutritional considerations should focus on balanced nutrition, not just increased calories (see Chapter 6).

Which CAM therapies are available to treat this condition?

Successful conventional interventions are available to treat aspects of this syndrome, such as vitamin A and amino acids. CAM therapy options such as omega-3 fatty acids, bee pollen, DHEA, licorice, soy supplements, and cyproheptadine may be helpful to some.

Are any CAM therapies being studied for this condition?

Wormwood is an approved herbal medicine for the treatment of reduced appetite in Germany. A U.S. study is under way to observe the helpful effects of wormwood supplementation in various chronic conditions, such as cancer, that are associated with reduced appetite.

ANXIETY

What is anxiety?

Anxiety is one of the most common psychological (emotional and mental) responses to the cancer experience. Anxiety may be felt while undergoing a cancer screening or diagnostic test, waiting for test results, receiving a cancer diagnosis, undergoing cancer treatment, or anticipating a cancer recurrence. Feelings of anxiety increase or decrease at different times, and the level of anxiety experienced by one person may differ from that experienced by another.

Anxiety associated with cancer can increase pain, cause insomnia (difficulty falling asleep or remaining asleep) or nausea and vomiting, and interfere with quality of life. For those patients with a history of an anxiety disorder that preceded their cancer diagnosis, anxiety can become overwhelming and potentially interfere with cancer treatment.

Which CAM therapies are available to treat this condition?

Kava has been used to help people fall asleep and fight fatigue, as well as to treat anxiety, insomnia, and menopausal symptoms. However, the U.S. Food and Drug Administration has issued a warning that use of kava supplements has been linked to a risk of severe liver damage.

Chamomile may be helpful for some people with mild to moderate generalized anxiety disorder. The chamomile extracts and formulations (oil or tea) might produce different results.

Other CAM therapies may have some benefit as well. Self-hypnosis and empathic attention reduced pain and anxiety during a breast biopsy for women. Cognitive-behavioral therapy may be useful in treating anxiety. The cognitive part helps people to change the thinking patterns that support their fears, and the behavioral part helps them to change the way they react to situations that produce anxiety.

Are any CAM therapies being studied for this condition?

Swedish massage or light touch is being studied for the treatment of generalized anxiety disorder. Chamomile extract therapy is under study to determine the long-term benefits for the prevention of recurrent anxiety disorder.

COGNITIVE DYSFUNCTION

What is cognitive dysfunction?

Cognitive dysfunction is described as difficulty with thinking ability, including memory loss, distractibility, difficulty in multitasking, and difficulty with arithmetic and language skills. Researchers note the difference between acute neurologic impairment and what is referred to as *chemobrain*, or problems with thinking and memory often experienced by people receiving chemotherapy. Mild to moderate cognitive dysfunction has been confirmed in patients receiving chemotherapy to treat cancer. Changes in thinking can have a significant impact on patients' quality of life.

Generally, chemotherapy does not cross the barrier between the bloodstream and the brain, which is referred to as the blood-brain barrier. Exceptions include carmustine, cisplatin, cytarabine, ifosfamide, lomustine, methotrexate, procarbazine, temozolomide, and topotecan.

Which CAM therapies are available to treat this condition?

There is no strong evidence to support the use of any CAM therapy for the prevention or treatment of cognitive dysfunction.

Are any CAM therapies being studied for this condition?

Research is needed to identify patients who are vulnerable to cognitive dysfunction from chemotherapy and the CAM therapies most likely to support traditional therapies in the prevention of or rehabilitation from cognitive dysfunction.

Aerobic exercise is being studied as an intervention to treat cancer-associated cognitive dysfunction. Tests that measure working memory, learning, and problem solving and functional magnetic resonance imaging will be used.

In a study conducted at West Virginia School of Medicine, one group of rats received two common cancer drugs, doxorubicin (Adriamycin®) and cyclophosphamide (Cytoxan®), four times weekly. Compared to the control animals, the rats that received chemotherapy had lower memory scores, indicating chemobrain. When rats received antioxidant N-acetylcysteine (NAC) injections three times weekly during chemotherapy, chemobrain was prevented. However, this intervention has not been tested in humans.

CONSTIPATION

What is constipation?

Constipation is a disorder characterized by the irregular and infrequent or difficult movement of the bowels. Cancer-related causes of constipation are mechanical pressure on the bowel (tumor, ascites [extra fluid in the stomach wall]), medications (chemotherapy, opioids), neurologic effects (pressure on the spinal cord), hypercalcemia, brachytherapy for gynecologic or prostate cancer (internal radiation therapy), and depression.

Other factors that can cause constipation include anorexia-cachexia syndrome, difficulty swallowing, inflammation of the mouth or digestive tract, and poorly controlled nausea and vomiting.

Which CAM therapies are available to treat this condition?

Flaxseed is a common CAM therapy used as a laxative. It contains soluble fiber, like that found in oat bran, and may have a laxative effect. Flaxseed oil comes from flaxseeds and is available in health food stores.

Several other CAM therapies are being used to treat constipation, such as aloe, barley, black psyllium, cascara, European buckthorn, glycerol, iodine, magnesium, olive oil, phosphorus, probiotics, and senna.

Are any CAM therapies being studied for this condition?

New cancer CAM studies are under way, but not for this symptom at the time of printing.

DEPRESSION

What is depression?

Depression is an illness that involves the body, mood, and thoughts. Depression affects the way a person eats and sleeps, the way one feels about oneself, and the way one thinks about life situations.

The incidence of depression in people with cancer is considerably higher than in the general population. Individuals and families who face a cancer diagnosis will experience varying levels of stress and emotional upset.

Which CAM therapies are available to treat this condition?

The most common CAM therapy for the treatment of depression is St. John's wort. Several other CAM therapies used to treat depression are art therapy, hypnosis and hypnotherapy, music therapy, and yoga.

Are any CAM therapies being studied for this condition?

Exercise therapy and cognitive-behavioral therapy are being studied for depression at this time.

DIARRHEA

What is diarrhea?

Diarrhea is a disorder characterized by frequent and watery bowel movements. Most cases of acute diarrhea have an abrupt onset, last for one to two weeks, have an infectious cause, and are self-limiting. Severe and uncontrolled diarrhea can lead to skin alterations with secondary infections, dehydration, electrolyte imbalance, and renal acid-base balance alterations.

Diarrhea commonly occurs in patients with cancer. Cancer-related causes of diarrhea can be associated with the disease or its treatment. Examples are certain tumors (lymphoma and colorectal), colitis, enzyme insufficiency, or infections (*Clostridium difficile*, cytomegalovirus). Examples of treatment-related causes are certain surgical procedures (colon resection, gastrectomy), chemotherapeutic agents, radiation to the abdomen or pelvis, or supportive care interventions (tube feedings, antibiotics).

Which CAM therapies are available to treat this condition?

Initial treatment for diarrhea is a clear liquid diet that includes water, weak tea, apple juice, clear broth, and gelatin with no solid foods. Probiotics (*Lactobacillus*), psyllium, and soy are common CAM therapies used to treat diarrhea.

Are any CAM therapies being studied for this condition?

Lactobacillus reuteri in oil droplet form is being studied for the prevention and treatment of mild diarrhea associated with gastrointestinal tract infections, travel, or antibiotic treatment.

FATIGUE

What is fatigue?

Cancer-related fatigue is the most common symptom reported by patients during cancer treatment. It is defined as a distressing, persistent sense of physical or emotional tiredness or exhaustion. The fatigue related to cancer or cancer treatment is not proportional to recent activity and interferes with usual functioning. It may occur alone or clustered with other symptoms.

The causes of fatigue in patients with cancer have not been determined, and management approaches vary. The focus of medical management often is directed at identifying specific and potentially reversible correlated symptoms (for example, anemia). Much of the information regarding interventions for fatigue relates either to healthy people or to fatigue as secondary to treatment-related anemia. Some recommendations for the management of fatigue in patients with cancer have been made, but with the exception of exercise, these are mostly theoretical and have not been the focus of scientific evaluation until recently.

Which CAM therapies are available to treat this condition?

Early intervention for fatigue includes balancing rest and activities, planning activities for when you have the most energy, planning enough rest and sleep, and taking short naps.

Very few CAM therapies have demonstrated strong evidence for the treatment of fatigue. Therapies that may be helpful are cognitive-behavioral therapy, ginseng, mild exercise, Reiki, and yoga.

Are any CAM therapies being studied for this condition?

Acupuncture combined with patient education is being studied to relieve fatigue in patients who have completed primary treatment for breast cancer.

HORMONAL CHANGES AND HOT FLASHES

What are hormonal changes and hot flashes?

Menopause is defined as the cessation of menstrual cycles for 12 consecutive months. Symptom severity varies. An early sign is irregular menses. As estrogen levels decline, insomnia, headaches, joint pain, vaginal dryness, tiredness, anxiety, irritability, mood swings, depression, loss of libido and memory, and concentration difficulties can occur with a range of severity and intensity. Sweats and hot flashes are common in cancer survivors. The broad-based treatment options include hormonal agents, nonhormonal drugs, and diverse CAM therapies.

Sweats are considered to be part of the hot flash complex and are a common experience in menopause. Hot flashes occur in patients with breast cancer. Menopause in a patient with cancer may be caused by surgery, chemotherapy, radiation, or androgen (hormone) treatment. Causes of "male menopause" include orchiectomy (surgical removal of the testes) or use of gonadotropin-releasing hormone or estrogen. Tamoxifen, aromatase inhibitors, opioids, tricyclic antidepressants, and steroids also can cause sweats.

Despite advances in traditional and CAM therapies that may decrease the well-documented discomfort and quality-of-life impact associated with hormonal changes and hot flashes, much remains to be learned regarding safe and effective interventions in long-term survivors of childhood cancers and older adults, including older men with prostate cancer. The impact of soy and phytonutrients and other CAM therapies remains controversial.

Which CAM therapies are available to treat this condition?

Little high-quality scientific evidence exists about the effectiveness and long-term safety of CAM therapies for menopausal symptoms. Black cohosh, dong quai root, ginseng, kava, red clover, and soy were studied for the treatment of menopausal-related symptoms and may be helpful. Acupuncture, flaxseed, relaxation, sage, valerian, and vitamin E also may be helpful for some individuals.

Are any CAM therapies being studied for this condition?

Hypnosis, acupuncture, mindfulness-based stress reduction, and practiced breathing are currently under study for the relief of hot flashes in both men and women.

INSOMNIA

What is insomnia?

Insomnia is a disorder characterized by difficulty falling asleep or remaining asleep. It is often a symptom of another underlying condition or situational circumstances such as jet lag, shift work, stress, poor sleep habits, or use of stimulants such as caffeine or other drugs.

The four typical types are (a) difficulty falling asleep, (b) difficulty maintaining sleep, (c) early morning awakening, and (d) unrefreshing sleep. All types can cause daytime sleepiness and potentially decrease productivity and increase the risk of accidents.

Which CAM therapies are available to treat this condition?

Strong evidence exists for the use of melatonin for the relief of jet lag. Acupuncture, aromatherapy, chamomile tea, cognitive-behavioral therapy, music therapy, self-hypnosis, and valerian also may be helpful.

Are any CAM therapies being studied for this condition?

Acupuncture, sleep directed hypnosis, and yoga are currently under study for the treatment of insomnia.

MUCOSITIS

What is mucositis?

Mucositis is a disorder characterized by inflammation of the oral mucosa, which is the lining of the mouth including the lips and upper and lower gums. Mucositis commonly occurs in patients who are treated with chemotherapy or radiation therapy. Following chemotherapy, mucositis most often develops in the small intestine but also occurs in the esophagus, stomach, and large intestine. Radiation esophagitis (irritation of the lining of the esophagus) and radiation proctitis (irritation of the lining of the rectum or anus) are forms of mucositis.

Mucositis not only produces discomfort and pain but also can lead to poor nutrition, delays in treatment, and increased hospital stays and costs. It first appears and often is most severe on the mucosa of the soft palate, tonsils, lining of the cheeks and lips, lateral border of the tongue, and walls of the throat.

Which CAM therapies are available to treat this condition?

There is no strong evidence to support the use of any CAM therapy for the prevention or treatment of mucositis. CAM therapies that may be helpful are acupuncture, chamomile, curcumin, glutamine, and Traumeel®.

Are any CAM therapies being studied for this condition?

Selenomethionine is being studied to reduce mucositis in patients with locally advanced head and neck cancer receiving chemotherapy and radiation. An oral rinse containing botanical extracts is being studied to prevent oral mucositis in patients with head and neck cancer receiving chemotherapy and radiation. A pilot study is under way to assess whether L-lysine may lessen the severity of oral mucositis in patients receiving radiation therapy with or without chemotherapy for head and neck cancer.

MYELOSUPPRESSION

What is myelosuppression?

Myelosuppression is a decrease in the production of red blood cells, white blood cells, and platelets in the bone marrow that are sent to the bloodstream on a constant basis. Decreases in these cell types can cause anemia, neutropenia, and thrombocytopenia.

Specifically, anemia is a reduction in the amount of hemoglobin within the bloodstream. Anemia may lead to dyspnea and fatigue. Neutropenia is a reduction in the amount of mature white blood cells, which may lead to an increased risk of infection. Thrombocytopenia is a reduction in the amount of platelets, which may lead to oozing, bruising, and bleeding.

Which CAM therapies are available to treat this condition?

Strong evidence exists for the treatment of anemia with vitamins and supplements such as folate, iron, vitamin B_{12}, vitamin B_6, and zinc. Liver extract and zinc also may be helpful for the treatment of anemia.

There is a lack of evidence for the use of CAM therapies for the treatment of decreased white blood cells and platelets.

Are any CAM therapies being studied for this condition?

New cancer CAM studies are under way, but not for this symptom at the time of printing.

NAUSEA AND VOMITING

What is nausea and vomiting?

Nausea is a disorder characterized by a queasy sensation and the urge to vomit. Vomiting is the act of expelling the contents of the stomach through the mouth. Nausea and vomiting commonly occur in patients with cancer. Nausea is considered to be a more frequent and perhaps more significant problem because it is underassessed and not as well controlled as vomiting.

Which CAM therapies are available to treat this condition?

Strong evidence is available to support the use of acupuncture for chemotherapy-related nausea and vomiting. Other CAM therapies that may be helpful are acustimulation, ginger, guided imagery, hypnosis, and music therapy.

Are any CAM therapies being studied for this condition?

Acupressure is being studied for its ability to reduce acute and delayed chemotherapy-related nausea and vomiting in pediatric patients with a variety of cancers.

Two dose levels of ginger are being compared in a study for patients undergoing chemotherapy who have experienced at least one episode of nausea and vomiting despite conventional therapy.

PAIN

What is cancer-related pain?

Pain can be a common occurrence in people with cancer. Most patients experience some level of pain during the cancer experience. Pain is considered the most feared of all symptoms associated with cancer. When pain is not relieved, it can affect all aspects of an individual's life. Pain contributes to suffering and has an overall negative effect on quality of life.

Specific cancer-related causes of pain include the presence of the tumor, a result of therapy, and prior or current painful conditions (e.g., arthritis). Pain can exist in several different forms, including acute versus chronic, neuropathic versus nociceptive, somatic, visceral, or psychogenic. Barriers to good management include misconceptions about the pain experience and pain medications.

Which CAM therapies are available to treat this condition?

Strong evidence exists for the use of massage for the treatment of pain. Other CAM therapies that may be helpful are distraction, guided imagery, hypnotherapy/hypnosis, music therapy, physical therapy, therapeutic touch, and relaxation.

Are any CAM therapies being studied for this condition?

Massage, meditation, and tai chi are under comparison in a study for the treatment of chronic lower back pain. The participants are assigned to one of the three interventions.

A pilot study is under way to test the effectiveness of CAM therapies and conventional care in patients with lower back pain. Following the evaluation, the two clinicians will meet and develop a treatment plan, which will include conventional medical care and some form of CAM such as acupuncture, chiropractic, exercise, massage, mind-body therapy, or nutritional counseling.

TASTE CHANGES

What are taste changes?

Taste changes are an abnormal shift in the taste of food and beverages. It can be described as *bad, me-*

tallic, salty, foul, or *rancid.* Because taste and smell are closely associated with eating, it is not clear whether these changes happen as a result of the changes in perception of smell or taste. Taste changes may be related to the site of the tumor, the extent of the tumor, the cancer therapy. Both perceptions are impaired temporarily and can be regenerated in most patients. Numerous self-help interventions are available to alleviate the severity but not the duration of taste changes in patients undergoing chemotherapy and radiation therapy.

Which CAM therapies are available to treat this condition?

No CAM therapies have shown strong evidence for the treatment of taste changes. Delta-9-tetrahydrocannabinol may be helpful for some individuals with taste changes because it may improve appetite as well.

Are any CAM therapies being studied for this condition?

New cancer CAM studies are under way, but not for this symptom at the time of printing.

XEROSTOMIA

What is xerostomia?

Xerostomia is the sensation of a dry mouth, usually as the result of decreased volume of secreted saliva or a change in the thickness of saliva. Patients undergoing treatment for cancer often report experiencing dry mouth. Salivary gland changes apply to both xerostomia and salivary gland hypofunction; both are side effects of radiation therapy to the head and neck region. It develops soon after radiation therapy begins, progresses, and is essentially permanent. Among the symptoms associated with reduced salivary function are oral discomfort, taste changes, difficulty chewing and swallowing, speech changes, dental decay, and oral candidiasis, a fungal infection.

Which CAM therapies are available to treat this condition?

There are no CAM therapies that have shown strong evidence for the treatment of xerostomia.

Are any CAM therapies being studied for this condition?

Acupuncture alone and in combination is under review in several studies for the treatment of xerostomia. Combination studies include acupuncture (specifically acupuncture-like transcutaneous electrical nerve stimulation) plus an effective treatment versus acupuncture alone.

WHAT IF I ALSO HAVE . . .

Allergies or Sensitivities to Certain Food

Food sensitivities and allergies may show as symptoms milder than or different from what we typically consider an allergy. Indigestion, headaches, cough, congestion, rashes, itching, sinus symptoms, joint pain, and other symptoms can alert you to a food sensitivity. Keeping a food/symptom journal can assist you in identifying food sensitivities. The most common food allergies/sensitivities include corn, eggs, dairy (milk), peanut, soy, shellfish, wheat, and yeast. Frequent allergens include apple, bacon, bean (dried), beef, berry, buckwheat, carrot, cheese, chocolate, cinnamon, coconut, coffee, fish, grape, mustard, nuts, onion, orange (citrus), pea, pork, potato, raisin, rye, shrimp, and tomato. The "Food Families" section outlines groups of foods that can have similar allergic properties. If you have food allergies, you must consider that any CAM therapy you use for allergies can potentially interfere with your cancer therapy.

FOOD FAMILIES

Certain foods are so similar that sensitivities to one food can create sensitivities to another. This is important because people often react to that "relative" of the food to which they are intolerant. For instance, if you are allergic or sensitive to oranges, you may also be allergic or sensitive to grapefruit. In the case of the grass family, a family to which most cereals belong, we consider subdivisions. The following groupings can help you identify foods to which you may have a sensitivity.

Food Family	Related Foods
Algae	Agar, dulse, kelp
Apple	Pear, quince, loquat, pectin, cider
Arum	Dasheen, eddoe
Aster	Lettuce, endive, globe and Jerusalem artichoke, dandelion, sunflower, tarragon, chamomile, yarrow, safflower oil
Banana	Plantain, arrowroot
Beech	Chestnut
Beef	Veal, all cow's milk products
Beet	Sugar beet, spinach, swiss chard, all beets, quinoa
Birch	Filbert, hazelnut, birch oil (wintergreen)
Bird	All fowl and game birds, including chicken, turkey, duck, goose, pigeon, quail, pheasant, partridge, grouse, all eggs
Blueberry	Bilberry, cranberry

(Continued on next page)

(Continued)

Food Family	Related Foods
Buckwheat	Amaranth, rhubarb, sorrell
Cashew	Mango, pistachio
Cereal (A)	Barley, bulgur, gluten, malt, rye, triticale, wheat, bran, wheat germ, graham
Cereal (B)	Oat
Cereal (C)	Corn, millet
Cereal (D)	Rice, wild rice
Cereal (E)	Bamboo shoot, sugarcane, molasses, sorghum
Citrus	Mandarin, grapefruit, kumquat, lemon, lime, orange, tangerine, citron
Composite	Artichoke, chamomile, chicory, dandelion, endive, escarole, head lettuce, leaf lettuce, safflower, tarragon
Conifer	Juniper, pine nut
Freshwater fish (A)	Herring, sardine, shad
Freshwater fish (B)	Pike, muskie (muskellunge)
Freshwater fish (C)	Salmon, trout
Freshwater fish (D)	Smelt
Freshwater fish (E)	Sturgeon, caviar
Freshwater fish (F)	Sunfish, black bass, bluegill, crappie
Fungus	Cheese (all), mushroom, sourdough, vinegar, all yeast
Ginger	Cardamom, ginger, turmeric, East Indian arrowroot
Goat	All goat products
Gooseberry	Currant, gooseberry
Goosefoot	Beet, beet sugar, lamb's-quarter, swiss chard, spinach

(Continued on next page)

(Continued)

Food Family	Related Foods
Gourd	Cantaloupe, casaba, cucumber, honeydew, all melons, pumpkin and seed, all squash, vegetable marrow, watermelon, zucchini
Grape	Grapes, raisin, wine, cream of tartar
Grass	Bamboo shoots, corn, oats, barley, kamut, malt, millet, rice, rye, spelt, sorghum, sugarcane, wheat
Heath	Blueberry, cranberry
Honeysuckle	Elderberry
Lamb	Mutton
Laurel	Avocado, bay leaves, cinnamon
Legumes	Alfalfa beans and sprouts, carob, chickpeas, fenugreek, kidney beans, lecithin, lentils, licorice, lima beans, mung beans, navy beans, all dried peas, pinto beans, peanuts, soybeans, split peas, string beans, tamarind, tofu
Lily	Asparagus, chive, garlic, leek, onion, shallot
Mallow	Okra, cottonseed
Maple	Sugar, syrup
Melon	Acorn squash and other squashes, cantaloupe, cucumber, honeydew, marrow, pumpkin, watermelon, zucchini
Mint	Apple mint, basil, bergamot, hyssop, lavender, lemon balm, marjoram, mint, oregano, peppermint, rosemary, sage, savory, spearmint, thyme
Moose	Venison
Mulberry	Breadfruit, fig, hop, mulberry

(Continued on next page)

(Continued)

Food Family	Related Foods
Mustard	Bok choy, broccoli, brussels sprout, cabbage, cauliflower, collard, horseradish, kale, kohlrabi, mustard/mustard seed, radish, rapeseed, rutabaga, salad mustard and cress, sprouts, turnip, watercress
Morning glory	Sweet potato
Myrtle	Allspice, clove, guava
Nutmeg	Mace
Olive	Black or green olives, olive oil
Palm	Coconut, date, date sugar, sago
Parsley	Anise, caraway, carrot, celery, celery root, coriander, cilantro, chervil, cumin, dill, fennel, lovage, parsley, parsnip
Pea	Dried beans, carob, fava beans, fenugreek, green beans, lentils, licorice, peanuts, red clover, senna, soybeans
Pepper	Black and white pepper, peppercorn
Pineapple	Pineapple
Plum	Almond, apricot, cherry, nectarine, peach, prune
Porcine	Bacon, ham, pork
Potato	Cayenne, chili pepper, eggplant, green pepper, paprika, red pepper, tobacco, tomato
Rose	Blackberry, loganberry, raspberry, rosehip, strawberry
Saltwater fish (A)	Anchovy
Saltwater fish (B)	Cod, haddock
Saltwater fish (C)	Flounder, halibut, sole, turbot
Saltwater fish (D)	Mackerel, tuna

(Continued on next page)

(Continued)

Food Family	Related Foods
Saltwater fish (E)	Red snapper
Saltwater fish (crustaceans)	Crab, crayfish, lobster, prawn, shrimp
Saltwater fish (mollusks)	Abalone, clam, mussel, oyster, scallop, squid
Spurge	Cassava, tapioca
Sterculia	Cocoa, cola, chocolate
Subucaya	Brazil nut
Sunflower	Jerusalem artichoke, sunflower oil, sunflower seed
Swine	All pork products
Tea	Green tea, pekoe tea
Walnut	Butternut, hickory nut, pecan, pineapple, pine nut, pomegranate, poppy seed, quinoa, saffron, sesame oil and seed, sweet potato/yam, taro root, vanilla

What CAM therapies are available to treat this condition?

- Scientific Evidence for Efficacy: low-allergen diet to reduce symptoms (sometimes used as a diagnostic tool), prevention/avoidance, reading food labels
- Conflicting Scientific Evidence: acupuncture, applied kinesiology, probiotics, *Lactobacillus acidophilus* (dairy free), thymus extract
- Insufficient or No Scientific Evidence: None

Are there any special pediatric or older adult considerations?

- Pediatrics: Pediatric food allergies/intolerances can be life threatening. Children with food allergies should be assessed by a specialist. Most CAM therapies have not been tested fully in the pediatric population to determine safety and efficacy. Safety regarding the use of these herbs and natural products in children is not known.
- Older adults: Older adults with food sensitivities respond best to avoidance of the food. The possibility of food sensitivities increases with age. As with the pediatric population, many CAM therapies have not been tested in the older adult population.

Chronic Obstructive Pulmonary Disease, Emphysema, or Asthma

Chronic obstructive pulmonary disease (COPD) is a lung disease that makes it difficult to breathe. There are two main forms of COPD: chronic bronchitis (a long-term cough with mucus) and emphysema, which involves damage to the lungs over time. Asthma, another form of airway disease, causes the airways of the lungs to swell, which leads to wheezing, shortness of breath, chest tightness, and coughing. Asthma symptoms can be triggered by breathing in allergy-causing substances called *allergens*, sometimes referred to as *triggers* (examples include dust and pet hair). The first step in addressing any therapy is to discontinue any use of tobacco. If you have COPD, you must consider that any CAM therapy you use can potentially interfere with your cancer therapy.

Any "attack" that threatens your ability to breathe is an emergency and requires immediate intervention. CAM therapies work slowly over a period of days to weeks.

What CAM therapies are available to treat these conditions?

- Scientific Evidence for Efficacy: Some trials demonstrated symptom reduction using *Radix glycyrrhizae* (licorice root) and an herbal formula called ASHMI (antiasthma herbal medicine intervention) with the drug prednisone in adults. Clinical results also were seen in patients with asthma taking *Sophora flavescens* Ait (a component of ASHMI).
- Conflicting Scientific Evidence: Boswellia should be avoided if you have a history of stomach ulcers or gastroesophageal reflux disease. Use with caution if taking sedatives, cholesterol-lowering-medications, or any agents metabolized by the liver's cytochrome P450 enzymes; if you have impaired liver function, liver damage, or lung disorders; and in children. Choline should be avoided if you are allergic or hypersensitive to choline, lecithin, or phosphatidylcholine; caution is required in those with kidney or liver disorders or trimethylaminuria and history of depression. Family psychotherapy has been found to be especially effective in decreasing wheezing in children. Buteyko breathing technique is an additional therapy with conflicting evidence for efficacy.
- Insufficient or No Scientific Evidence: Evening primrose oil, lycopene, L-arginine, reflexology, vitamin E

Are there any special pediatric or older adult considerations?

- Pediatrics: Three clinical trials using specific herbal formulas have been tested in asthmatic children, and a reduction of symptoms has been seen. Most CAM therapies have not been tested fully in the pediatric population to determine safety and efficacy. Further study is needed to determine safety regarding use of these herbs and natural products in children.

- Older adults: The shortness of breath that accompanies COPD and emphysema can cause an elder to become depressed, anxious, and frightened whether living alone or in a group. It can interfere with nutrition, socialization, and the ability to tolerate cancer therapy.

Diabetes

Diabetes is an error in glucose metabolism. Two types of diabetes exist: type 1 and type 2. Having diabetes can cause concern for the person's nutritional status and other issues during cancer treatment. If you have diabetes, you must consider that any CAM therapy you use for diabetes can potentially interfere with your cancer therapy.

What CAM therapies are available to treat this condition?

- Scientific Evidence for Efficacy: Alpha lipoic acid should be used cautiously in diabetes and thyroid diseases and avoided if you are allergic to alpha lipoic acid or have thiamine deficiency or alcoholism. American ginseng has evidence of efficacy, but in individuals with type 2 diabetes and hyperglycemia, it may increase the effects of blood sugar–lowering medications, including insulin. Avoid this agent if you have a known allergy to plants in the *Araliaceae* family because of the risk for a life-threatening skin reaction. Beta-glucan, which is usually used for cholesterol-lowering effects, is now also used for glycemic (blood sugar) control in people with diabetes. Avoid beta-glucan if you are allergic or hypersensitive to beta-glucan, and people with AIDS or AIDS-related complex should exercise caution with it. Chromium has evidence of efficacy but should be avoided if you are allergic to chromium, chromate, or leather. It should be used with caution if you have depression, diabetes, liver problems, or a weakened immune system or are an organ transplant recipient. Caution is also necessary if you have Parkinson disease, heart disease, or stroke and are taking medications for one of these conditions, and if you are driving or operating machinery. Exercise and weight control have shown efficacy in the treatment of diabetes. Gymnema may increase the effects of blood sugar–lowering medications, including insulin; therefore, avoid using it with medications that lower blood sugar. Magnesium and whey protein (caution if you take any medications) also have evidence for their use in diabetes.

- Conflicting Scientific Evidence: acupuncture, alfalfa, aloe vera, arabinoxylan, ashwagandha, astragalus, Atkins diet, barley, beets, bilberry, biotin, bitter melon, black tea, burdock root or fruit, CoQ10, chrysanthemum, cinnamon, dandelion, evening primrose oil, fig, flaxseed, garlic, glucosamine, green tea, holy basil, honey, hydrotherapy, jackfruit, kudzu, L-carnitine, lutein, maitake, massage, milk thistle, myrcia, niacin, nopal (prickly pear), omega-3 fatty acids, onion, psychotherapy, psyllium, qigong, red clover, red yeast rice, reflexology, Reishi mushrooms, safflower, seaweed, selenium, soy, spirulina, stevia, tai chi, therapeutic touch, thymus extract, vitamin D, vitamin E, white horehound, yoga, zinc
- Insufficient or No Scientific Evidence: CoQ10, prayer, selenium

Are there any special pediatric or older adult considerations?

Trials have not evaluated the use of these therapies in children or older adults; therefore, there is insufficient information regarding their safety and efficacy in these populations.

Headaches

Do not use any self-prescribed therapy if your headaches are accompanied by vision changes, nausea, or temporal artery pain or if you have a history of blood clot or stroke and have not been assessed by your healthcare provider. If you have headaches, you must consider that any CAM therapy you use for headaches can potentially interfere with your cancer therapy.

• Scientific Evidence for Efficacy: Feverfew has evidence for its use, but avoid if you are allergic to chrysanthemums, daisies, marigold, or ragweed. 5-HTP has shown efficacy but should not be used if you are taking antidepressants or in doses that exceed those recommended. Arginine can be considered, but avoid if you have a history of allergy to arginine, kidney or liver disease, or sickle-cell disease or if you are on diabetes medications. Serum potassium levels should be monitored. Butterbur is another agent to consider unless you are allergic to the aster family: chrysanthemums, asters, marigolds, and daisies. Chiropractic, guided imagery, hypnotherapy, and peppermint (except in gallbladder disease or G6PD deficiency) also have shown evidence of efficacy.

• Conflicting Scientific Evidence: acupuncture, acupressure, belladonna, black cohosh, capsicum, CoQ10, dong quai, eucalyptus oil, gamma-linolenic

acid, ginger, massage, niacin, shiatsu, soy, tai chi, vitamin B_2 (riboflavin), willow bark
- Insufficient or No Scientific Evidence: L-arginine, melatonin, progressive muscle relaxation, reflexology

Are there any special pediatric or older adult considerations?

Trials have not evaluated the use of these therapies in children or older adults; therefore, there is insufficient information regarding their safety and efficacy in these populations.

Heart Disease

Heart disease is the term used to describe conditions that affect the heart muscle or the blood vessels of the heart. High cholesterol and high blood pressure can lead to heart disease and will be considered in this section. Many different types of heart disease exist. The most common is coronary artery disease (also known as CAD). This condition can cause the arteries to narrow, leading to an increased risk for a stroke or heart attack. If you have heart disease, you must consider that any CAM therapy you use for heart disease may have the potential to interfere with your cancer therapy.

- Scientific Evidence for Efficacy
  - Beta glucan
  - Beta stilbestrol (potential for many drug reactions including those used in cancer treatment)
  - Calcium—Avoid if allergic or hypersensitive to calcium or lactose. Oral calcium in high doses may cause kidney stones. Avoid if you have or have had hypercalcemia (high levels of calcium in the

blood), hypercalciuria (high levels of calcium in urine), hyperparathyroidism (high levels of para-thyroid hormone), bone tumors, digitalis toxici-ty, ventricular fibrillation, history of kidney stones, kidney disease, or sarcoidosis. Dangerous levels of lead have been found in calcium supplements made from dolomite, oyster shells, or bone meal; use only under medical supervision with absence or low levels of hydrochloric acid in gastric juices (achlorhydria), arrhythmia (irregular heartbeat), or certain cancers.

– Niacin—Use with caution and only under medical supervision because of the early ability of niacin to promote collateral circulation to a tumor.

– Omega-3 fatty acids to reduce triglyceride levels— Avoid if allergic or hypersensitive to fish, omega-3 fatty acid products that come from fish, nuts, or linolenic acid or omega-3 fatty acid products that come from nuts. Avoid during active bleeding; medical supervision is needed with a diagnosis of a bleeding disorders, diabetes, or low blood pres-sure or if taking drugs, herbs, or supplements that treat any such conditions. Avoid for at least 10 days to two weeks before surgery.

– Red yeast rice—Avoid if allergic or hypersensitive to red yeast and with liver disease.

– Soy—High doses of soy or soy isoflavones are not recommended for anyone. Those with intestinal ir-ritation from cow's milk may experience intestinal damage or diarrhea from soy. Use is discouraged in patients with hormone-sensitive cancers, such as breast, ovarian, or uterine cancer. Hormone-sensi-tive conditions (e.g., endometriosis) may worsen. Avoid if taking blood-thinners like warfarin.

- Arginine has shown improvement in blood flow in those with coronary artery disease, but safe doses have not yet been established. Avoid if allergic to arginine; with a history of stroke or liver or kidney disease; use only under medical supervision if taking blood-thinning drugs, drugs to control blood sugar, or herbs or supplements with similar effect; may worsen symptoms of sickle-cell disease.
- Garlic to lower total cholesterol and LDL cholesterol—Avoid if allergic or hypersensitive to garlic or other members of the *Lilaceae* (lily) family, such as hyacinth, tulip, onion, leek, or chive. Avoid with history of bleeding problems; on blood thinning drugs; or with asthma, diabetes, low blood pressure, or thyroid disorders. Discontinue use at least two weeks before dental, surgical, or diagnostic procedures and after these procedures (check with your healthcare provider) to avoid bleeding problems.

• Conflicting Scientific Evidence: Acupuncture should be avoided if you have valvular heart disease, infections, or a bleeding disorder or if you are taking drugs that increase the risk of bleeding (anticoagulants). You should also avoid it if you have undiagnosed medical conditions or neurologic disorders, areas that have received radiation therapy, or pulmonary disease such as asthma or emphysema. Older adults, medically compromised individuals, people with diabetes, and those with a history of seizures should not undergo acupuncture. Avoid electroacupuncture if you have arrhythmia (irregular heartbeat) or a pacemaker. Astragalus is another therapy with conflicting evidence, and drug interactions are possible. Berberine use requires caution if you have cardiovascular disease, a gastrointestinal disorder, a hematologic disorder, leukopenia (low white blood cells), kidney disease, liver disease, a respiratory disorder, cancer, diabetes, or hypotension, and it has the potential to interact with numerous drugs. It should not be used in children, as no safety data exist. Biotin, black tea, DHEA, elderberry, fenugreek, ginkgo, ginseng, goldenseal, horny goat weed, *Lactobacillus acidophilus*, macrobiotic diet, peony, and turmeric are additional therapies with conflicting evidence.

- Insufficient or No Scientific Evidence: acacia, beta-carotene, glucosamine, relaxation therapy, vitamin C, vitamin E.

Are there any special pediatric or older adult considerations?

Trials have not evaluated the use of these therapies in children or older adults; therefore, there is insufficient information regarding their safety and efficacy in these populations.

CAM USE IN PEDIATRIC AND ADOLESCENT POPULATIONS

What is the use of CAM in pediatric and adolescent medicine?

CAM use in pediatric and adolescent medicine is increasing. Many patients are also receiving conventional therapies. These patients are more likely to be seeing their pediatrician for an illness or ongoing medical problems and taking medication regularly.

The use of CAM is higher in certain groups of children, such as those with special care needs, homeless adolescents, and those with chronic conditions such as asthma, rheumatoid arthritis, and cancer.

Parents may seek CAM therapies for their children because of word of mouth, media report of safe and effective therapies, fear of side effects from conventional therapies, and cultural values and beliefs.

What is the use of CAM in pediatric and adolescent oncology?

Cancer is the leading cause of death by disease in children between infancy and age 15. A 2010 review led by the American Academy of Pediatrics showed that between 6% and 91% of children with cancer use CAM at some point during their conventional therapy. The most common therapies used were herbal therapies, nutrition and diet therapies, and faith-healing. Homeopathy, megavitamins, mind-body therapies, and massage were also used. The reasons for CAM use were to cure or help fight the cancer and to provide symptom management.

Are there any special considerations for children and adolescents experiencing specific symptoms?

Clinicians have much to learn and research regarding CAM use in this population. Most CAM therapies have not been tested fully in these patients to determine safety and efficacy. Following are symptoms for which special pediatric considerstions are known to exist.

- Anxiety: Treatment of childhood cancer is a challenging and highly stressful experience for the child and the family. It is believed that children undergoing cancer treatment are at a higher risk for psychological distress, including depression and anxiety. There is evidence that children experience distress during the cancer treatment process. Distress appears to be most significant early in therapy, typically when frequent hospitalizations are necessary, with a pattern of less distress occurring over time.

- Depression: Most children cope with the emotional upheaval related to cancer and demonstrate not only evidence of adaptation but positive psychosocial growth and development. A minority of children develop psychological problems including depression, anxiety, sleep disturbances, difficulties in interpersonal relationships, and noncompliance with treatment. These children require referral and intervention by a mental health specialist.
- Fatigue: It is difficult to define, measure, and develop effective interventions for fatigue in children and adolescents with cancer. Fatigue in these patients exists within a greater context of illness, treatment, and development.
- Hormonal changes and hot flashes: Little is known about hot flashes in children with cancer. Hormonal changes are relative to the cancer site treated. Survivorship issues are being explored, and research is ongoing with long-term cancer survivors.
- Insomnia: Sleep disorders in children and teens are largely underdiagnosed. Children who snore, have problems falling asleep, are difficult to wake in the morning, or fall asleep in school should be further evaluated for sleep disorders.
- Mucositis: In children receiving chemotherapy, the incidence of oral mucositis is reported to be 52%–

80%. Oral infections and tooth decay during chemotherapy can be prevented with diligent oral care,
but this is challenging in this age group. New and effective therapies for the relief of mucositis are needed in this population.

• Myelosuppression: A child who has anemia may
not know it because he or she may not have any
symptoms. Possible symptoms include looking
pale, a fast heartbeat, and fatigue. The most common cause for anemia in children is lack of dietary iron. Adding iron-rich foods to the child's
diet will help.

Where can I find more information about CAM use in pediatrics and adolescents?

A number of groups across the United States promote research and inform the public about CAM use
in pediatric and adolescent patients with cancer. Some
examples are

• American Academy of Pediatrics Provisional Section
on Complementary and Integrative Medicine, www
.aap.org/sections/chim/default.cfm

• CureSearch for Children's Cancer, www.curesearch
.org

• National Cancer Institute Childhood Cancers, www
.cancer.gov/cancertopics/types/childhoodcancers

• Pediatric Complementary and Alternative Medicine
Research and Education Network, www.pedcam.ca

What can we anticipate for future research in this area?

Ongoing study challenges with CAM use include
determining efficacy and safety, mechanism of action, potential interactions, pediatric dosing, and cost-

effectiveness. Unique needs related to the pediatric and adolescent populations include finding trained practitioners with pediatric experience who have a complete understanding of sensitive patient outcome criteria across age groups and protecting risk and respecting autonomy with assent/consent considerations.

CAM USE IN OLDER ADULTS

What is the use of CAM in geriatric medicine?

The 65-and-older population is growing. By 2020, one in five adults will be older than age 65. For some older adults, this means living longer with pain and other symptoms. Surveys show that older adults use CAM therapies to provide relief, chiefly for age-related arthritis, back pain, headaches, and chronic pain.

A survey of 1,559 older adults showed that the top CAM therapies used were massage, movement therapy, bodywork, and dietary supplements and herbal products. Of the respondents, 63% used one or more CAM therapies.

What is the use of CAM in geriatric oncology?

The prevalence of CAM use in geriatric oncology is not well known. The American Cancer Society recently analyzed the prevalence and medical and demographic relationships between CAM use in 4,139 cancer survivors. The study revealed that more advanced age at diagnosis predicted a greater likelihood of CAM use and that the most frequently reported CAMs were prayer/spiritual practice, relaxation, and vitamins and supplements.

What are two main areas of focus in geriatric oncology?

Chemoprevention is a main focus area in this field. The leading sites for cancer mortality are cancers of the lung, pancreas, prostate, breast, and ovary and non-Hodgkin lymphoma. Some examples of cancer-fighting substances are cruciferous vegetables, resveratrol, green tea, and antioxidants.

The other main area of interest is **polypharmacy and interactions**. *Polypharmacy* is a newer term used to describe the use of many medications by one person. Sometimes, a patient may be taking more than one medication for the same condition. Older adults often take prescription drugs in combination with over-the-counter medicines and supplements. Many patients taking herbs and supplements fail to report this use to their healthcare providers. Among the CAM users in a recent study, more than half of all drug interactions identified were related to the CAM therapies.

Are there any special considerations for older adults experiencing specific symptoms?

Much is known, but much remains to be learned regarding CAM use in older adults. Following are symptoms for which special geriatric considerations are know to exist.
- Anorexia/cachexia: Anorexia may occur alongside dementia (changes in memory and mental function), depression, or cancer in older adults. Visual (eyesight) or sensory (hearing or feeling) problems, living alone, low income, lack of transportation, or living in a group setting can negatively affect nutrition.
- Anxiety: See Depression.

- Cognitive dysfunction: Changes in cognition were long thought to be an expected consequence of cancer treatment. Clinicians have much to learn about CAM therapies for cognitive impairment in older patients.
- Constipation: About 30% of adults age 65 and older have chronic constipation, with a greater incidence noted in women. Constipation may occur as a side effect of drugs or may be a manifestation of metabolic or neurologic disease. In all situations, colon obstruction must be ruled out. Constipation among patients with dementia is common, especially with the use of psychotropic medications. Patients may not always be relied upon to describe symptoms accurately, so healthcare providers should take a proactive approach.
- Depression: The incidence of depression is known to increase with age and has been associated with increased morbidities. Depression is one of the most frequent reasons for seeking CAM therapies, including St. John's wort, progressive muscle relaxation, music therapy, massage, exercise, aromatherapy, dance and movement therapy, and relaxation.
- Diarrhea: Additional causes of diarrhea may be fecal impaction, lactose intolerance, gastrointestinal conditions (irritable bowel syndrome, malabsorption, and inflammatory bowel disease), infections, or medications. Older adults have an increased risk of complications associated with diarrhea such as dehydration, altered drug metabolism, compromised cardiac status, and confusion.
- Fatigue: Fatigue in older patients with cancer has not been well studied. It will be affected by variables such as treatment, medical age of the patient, and the presence or absence of other illnesses.

- Hormonal changes and hot flashes: Little is known about hot flashes in this population. Survivorship issues are being explored, and research are ongoing with those who are long-term survivors.
- Insomnia: Older adults often have problems sleeping, including difficulty falling asleep, waking up during the night, and waking up very early in the morning. At least half of older adults use over-the-counter or prescription medications to help them sleep. Nonpharmacologic interventions are preferred for managing sleep problems. As long as older adults feel refreshed when they awaken, they are likely getting enough sleep. Providing a regular schedule of meals, discouraging daytime naps, and encouraging physical activity may improve sleep.
- Mucositis: Age-related changes such as decreased salivary flow, increased gingivitis, and decreased mucosal regeneration may contribute to an increased risk of severe oral and gastrointestinal mucositis.
- Myelosuppression: Anemia is the most common age-related blood-related abnormality in older men and women, and many tests fail to identify a cause. Anemia may increase the risk for adverse drug reactions, risk of delirium, and complications from chemotherapy. Thrombocytopenia is a common cause of bleeding problems in older adults and can present as unexplained bruises, nosebleeds, or gastrointestinal losses (increased bowel movements including diarrhea). Bleeding can occur when the platelet count drops to 20,000 per µL or less. Immune thrombocytopenia is usually a secondary presentation in older adults, so the initial approach is to identify and treat the primary cause.

- Nausea and vomiting: Evaluation and prompt intervention of nausea and vomiting is necessary if it is related to chemotherapy. If the patient is not seriously ill or dehydrated, assessment on an outpatient basis for spontaneous, non–treatment-related nausea or vomiting can possibly wait 24–48 hours. Older adults who are taking antinausea medicine have an increased risk of side effects and require close monitoring.
- Pain: Pain assessment may be more complex in the older adult because of multiple medical problems, cognitive impairment, underreporting of pain, misconceptions about pain events and pain management, multiple sources of pain, multiple medications with potential interactions, and alterations in how these medications are metabolized in the bloodstream.
- Taste changes: Older patients experience a reduction of taste sensation and olfactory function but not taste discrimination. For example, older adults may be able to distinguish sweet from salty but may need to add more salt to food to taste it completely.
- Xerostomia: Salivary function is not noticeably reduced with aging, but xerostomia can be a common complaint of older patients, usually because of the adverse effects of medication.

Where can I find more information about CAM use in older adults?

A number of groups across the United States provide information about CAM use in this population of patients with cancer, such as the following.

- AARP, www.aarp.org
- American Cancer Society, www.cancer.org

- American Geriatrics Society, www.americangeriatrics
  .org
- The Geriatric Oncology Consortium, www.thegoc
  .org
- National Institute on Aging, www.nia.nih.gov
- NIHSeniorHealth (National Institutes of Health),
  http://nihseniorhealth.gov

BIBLIOGRAPHY

AARP & National Center for Complementary and Alternative Medicine. (2007). *Complementary and alternative medicine: What people 50 and older are using and discussing with their physicians.* Retrieved from http://assets.aarp.org/rgcenter/health/cam_2007.pdf

A.D.A.M. (2011). Asthma—children. In *A.D.A.M. medical encyclopedia.* Retrieved from http://www.ncbi.nlm.nih.gov/pubmed health/PMH0001985

Ahles, T.A., & Saykin, A.J. (2001). Cognitive effects of standard-dose chemotherapy in patients with cancer. *Cancer Investigation, 19,* 812–820.

American Cancer Society. (2011a). Chemotherapy principles: An in-depth discussion: Taste changes. Retrieved from http://www.cancer.org/Treatment/TreatmentsandSideEffects/TreatmentTypes/Chemotherapy/index

American Cancer Society. (2011b). Fatigue. Retrieved from http://www.cancer.org/Treatment/TreatmentsandSideEffects/PhysicalSideEffects/DealingwithSymptomsatHome/caring-for-the-patient-with-cancer-at-home-fatigue

American Geriatrics Society. (2011). Palliative care. Retrieved from http://www.americangeriatrics.org

American Lung Association. (n.d.-a). Asthma. Retrieved from http://www.lungusa.org/lung-disease/asthma

American Lung Association. (n.d.-b). COPD. Retrieved from http://www.lungusa.org/lung-disease/copd

Balducci, L. (2003). Myelosuppression and its consequences in elderly patients with cancer. *Oncology, 17*(11, Suppl. 11), 27–32.

Balducci, L., & Beghe, C. (2004). Chemoprevention of cancer in the older person. In L. Balducci, G.H. Lyman, W.B. Ershler, & M. Extermann (Eds.), *Comprehensive geriatric oncology* (2nd ed., pp. 349–364). Abingdon, Oxon, UK: Taylor & Francis.

Balducci, L., & Corcoran, M.B. (2000). Antineoplastic chemotherapy of the older cancer patient. *Hematology/Oncology Clinics of
North America, 14,* 193–212. doi:10.1016/S0889-8588(05)70284-
7

Bishop, F.L., Prescott, P., Chan, Y.K., Saville, J., von Elm, E., &
Lewith, G.T. (2010). Prevalence of complementary medicine
use in pediatric cancer: A systematic review. *Pediatrics, 125,*
768–767. doi:10.1542/peds.2009-1775

Cheng, K.K.F., & Chang, A.M. (2003). Palliation of oral mucositis
symptoms in pediatric patients treated with cancer chemotherapy. *Cancer Nursing, 26,* 476–484.

Children's Hospital of New York-Presbyterian. (n.d.). The Integrative Therapies Program for Children with Cancer. Retrieved   from   http://integrativetherapies.columbia.edu/
MANUSCRIPT.html#bringingevidence

ClinicalTrials.gov. (2011a). Can exercise improve cancer associated cognitive dysfunction? (chemobrain). Retrieved from
http://www.clinicaltrials.gov/ct2/show/NCT01296893?term
=cognitive+dysfunction+AND+chemotherapy&rank=12

ClinicalTrials.gov. (2011b). Efficacy of massage therapy in the treatment of generalized anxiety disorder (GAD) (ClinicalTrials
.gov identifier: NCT01337713). Retrieved from http://www
.clinicaltrials.gov

ClinicalTrials.gov. (2011c). Hot flashes [Search results]. Retrieved August 21, 2011, from http://clinicaltrials.gov/ct2/
results?term=hot+flashes

ClinicalTrials.gov. (2011d). Insomnia and CAM [Search results].
Retrieved August 21, 2011, from http://clinicaltrials.gov/ct2/
results?term=insomnia+and+CAM

ClinicalTrials.gov. (2011e). Long-term chamomile therapy for
anxiety (ClinicalTrials.gov identifier: NCT01072344). Retrieved from http://www.clinicaltrials.gov

ClinicalTrials.gov. (2011f). Pain and CAM [Search results]. Retrieved August 21, 2011, from http://clinicaltrials.gov/ct2/
results?term=pain+and+CAM

ConsumerLab.com. (n.d.). Retrieved from http://www.consumerlab
.com

Decker, G. (2006). Complementary and alternative therapies. In
D. Cope & A. Reb (Eds.), *An evidence-based approach to the treatment and care of the older adult with cancer* (pp. 485–528). Pittsburgh, PA: Oncology Nursing Society.

Gansler, T., Kaw, C., Crammer, C., & Smith, T. (2008). A population-based study of prevalence of complementary methods
use by cancer survivors: A report from the American Cancer

Society's studies of cancer survivors. *Cancer, 113,* 1048–1057. doi:10.1002/cncr.23659

Gardner, N.M., & Cope, D.G. (2006). Symptom management of diarrhea and constipation. In D.G. Cope & A.M. Reb (Eds.), *An evidence-based approach to the treatment and care of the older adult with cancer* (pp. 367–389). Pittsburgh, PA: Oncology Nursing Society.

Henley, D.V., Lipson, N., Korach, K.S., & Bloch, C.A. (2007). Prepubertal gynecomastia linked to lavender and tea tree oils. *New England Journal of Medicine, 356,* 479–485. doi:10.1056/NEJ Moa064725

Jakobsen, J.N., & Herrstedt, J. (2009). Prevention of chemotherapy-induced nausea and vomiting in elderly cancer patients. *Critical Reviews in Oncology/Hematology, 71,* 214–221. doi:10.1016/j .critrevonc.2008.12.006

Jansen, C., Miaskowski, C., Dodd, M., Dowling, G., & Kramer, J. (2005). Potential mechanisms for chemotherapy-induced impairments in cognitive function. *Oncology Nursing Forum, 32,* 1151–1163. doi:10.1188/05.ONF.1151-1163

Kemper, K.J., Vohra, S., & Walls, R. (2008). The use of complementary and alternative medicine in pediatrics. *Pediatrics, 122,* 1374–1386. doi:10.1542/peds.2008-2173

Kennedy, B.J. (2004). Aging and cancer. In L. Balducci, G.H. Lyman, W.B. Ershler, & M. Extermann (Eds.), *Comprehensive geriatric oncology* (2nd ed., pp. 3–10). Abingdon, Oxon, UK: Taylor & Francis.

Lang, E.V., Berbaum, K.S., Faintuch, S., Hatsiopoulou, O., Halsey, N., Li, X., ... Baum, J. (2006). Adjunctive self-hypnotic relaxation for outpatient medical procedures: A prospective randomized trial with women undergoing large core breast biopsy. *Pain, 126,* 155–164. doi:10.1016/j.pain.2006.06.035

Lee, R.T., Qato, D., Curlin, F., Stadler, W.M., & Lindau, S.T. (2008). Older cancer survivors' use of biologically based complementary and alternative medicine (CAM): A national, population-based study in the United States. *Journal of Clinical Oncology, 26*(15S, May 20 Suppl.), Abstract 9508. Retrieved from http://meeting.ascopubs.org/cgi/content/abstract/26/15 _suppl/9508

Li, X.-M., & Brown, L.V. (2009). Efficacy and mechanisms of action of traditional Chinese medicines for treating asthma and allergy. *Journal of Allergy and Clinical Immunology, 123,* 297–306. doi:10.1016/j.jaci.2008.12.026

MedlinePlus. (2011a). Constipation. Retrieved from http://www .nlm.nih.gov/medlineplus/constipation.html#cat4

MedlinePlus. (2011b). Generalized anxiety disorder. Retrieved from http://www.nlm.nih.gov/medlineplus/ency/article/000917 .htm

Montalto, C.P., Bhargava, V., & Hong, G.S. (2006). Use of complementary and alternative medicine by older adults: An exploratory study. *Complementary Health Practice Review, 11*, 27–46. doi:10.1177/1533210106288823

Morris, P.B., Ellis, M.N., & Swain, J.L. (1989). Angiogenic potency of nucleotide metabolites: Potential role in ischemia-induced vascular growth. *Journal of Molecular and Cellular Cardiology, 21*, 351–358. doi:10.1016/0022-2828(89)90645-7

National Cancer Institute. (2011a). Clinical trials (PDQ®): Xerostomia acupuncture trial. Retrieved from http://www.cancer .gov/clinicaltrials/search/view?cdrid=692260&version=Healt hProfessional&protocolsearchid=9544802

National Cancer Institute. (2011b). Depression (PDQ®). Retrieved from http://www.cancer.gov/cancertopics/pdq/ supportivecare/depression/Patient

National Cancer Institute. (2011c). Improving fatigue: A pilot study of acupuncture and patient education for breast cancer survivors. Retrieved from http://www.cancer.gov/clinical trials/search/view?cdrid=593370&version=Patient&protocol searchid=6515675

National Cancer Institute. (2011d). L-lysine in treating oral mucositis in patients undergoing radiation therapy with or without chemotherapy for head and neck cancer. Retrieved from http://www.cancer.gov/clinicaltrials/search/view?cdrid=681 490&version=HealthProfessional&protocolsearchid=7728786

National Cancer Institute. (2011e). Nutrition in cancer care (PDQ®) [Health professional version]. Retrieved from http://www .cancer.gov/cancertopics/pdq/supportivecare/nutrition/ healthprofessional

National Cancer Institute. (2011f). Oral complications of chemotherapy and head/neck radiation (PDQ®): Taste dysfunction. Retrieved from http://www.cancer.gov/cancertopics/ pdq/supportivecare/oralcomplications/healthprofessional/ allpages#Section_329

National Cancer Institute. (2011g). Phase II/III randomized study of acupuncture-like transcutaneous electrical nerve stimulation (ALTENS) versus pilocarpine hydrochloride in head and neck cancer patients with early radiotherapy-induced xerostomia. Retrieved from http://www.cancer.gov/clinicaltrials/ search/view?cdrid=592644&version=HealthProfessional& protocolsearchid=9544802

National Cancer Institute. (2011h). Safety and efficacy of IZN-6N4 oral rinse for the prevention of oral mucositis in patients with head and neck cancer. Retrieved from http://www.cancer.gov/clinicaltrials/search/vie?cdrid=706757&version=Health Professional&protocolsearchid=7728786

National Cancer Institute. (2011i). Selenomethionine in reducing mucositis in patients with locally advanced head and neck cancer receiving cisplatin and radiation therapy. Retrieved from http://www.cancer.gov/clinicaltrials/search/view?cdrid=647 812&version=HealthProfessional&protocolsearchid=7728786

National Cancer Institute. (2011j). Sleep disorders. Retrieved from http://www.cancer.gov/cancertopics/pdq/supportivecare/sleepdisorders/Patient/page5

National Cancer Institute. (2011k). Wormwood in chronic progressive disorders with reduced appetite. Retrieved from http://www.cancer.gov/clinicaltrials/search/view?cdrid=674 230&version=HealthProfessional&protocolsearchid=9536918

National Center for Biotechnology Information. (n.d.-a). Asthma. Retrieved from http://www.ncbi.nlm.nih.gov

National Center for Biotechnology Information. (n.d.-b). Chronic obstructive pulmonary disease (COPD). Retrieved from http://www.ncbi.nlm.nih.gov

National Center for Complementary and Alternative Medicine. (2009a). Chinese herbal medicine may benefit people with prediabetes, but evidence is inconclusive. Retrieved from http://nccam.nih.gov/research/results/spotlight/110309.htm

National Center for Complementary and Alternative Medicine. (2009b). Study shows chamomile capsules ease anxiety symptoms. Retrieved from http://nccam.nih.gov/research/results/spotlight/040310.htm

National Center for Complementary and Alternative Medicine. (2010). Kava. Retrieved from http://nccam.nih.gov/health/kava

National Center for Complementary and Alternative Medicine. (2011a). Asthma. Retrieved from http://nccam.nih.gov/health/asthma

National Center for Complementary and Alternative Medicine. (2011b). Effects of chromium picolinate in people at risk for type 2 diabetes. Retrieved from http://nccam.nih.gov/research/results/spotlight/020111.htm

National Center for Complementary and Alternative Medicine. (2011c). Flaxseed and flaxseed oil. Retrieved from http://nccam.nih.gov/health/flaxseed/ataglance.htm

National Center for Complementary and Alternative Medicine. (2011d). Menopausal symptoms and CAM. Retrieved from http://nccam.nih.gov/health/menopause/menopause symptoms.htm

National Center for Complementary and Alternative Medicine. (2011e). Sleep disorders and CAM: At a glance. Retrieved from http://nccam.nih.gov/health/sleep/ataglance.htm

National Institute on Aging. (2011). Age page: Concerned about constipation? Retrieved from http://www.nia.nih.gov/Health Information/Publications/constipation.htm

Natural Medicines Comprehensive Database. (n.d.). Retrieved from http://naturaldatabase.therapeuticresearch.com

Natural Standard Research Collaboration. (n.d.). Retrieved from http://www.naturalstandard.com

Post-White, J., Hawks, R., O'Mara, A., & Ott, M.J. (2006). Future directions of CAM research in pediatric oncology. *Journal of Pediatric Oncology Nursing, 23*, 265–268. doi:10.1177/1043454206291361

Wilkes, G.M., & Barton-Burke, M. (2007). *Oncology nursing drug handbook.* Sudbury, MA: Jones and Bartlett.

Zebrack, B.J., Gurney, J.G., Oeffinger, K., Whitton, J., Packer, R.J., Mertens, A., ... Zeltzer, L.K. (2004). Psychological outcomes in long-term survivors of childhood brain cancer: A report from the childhood cancer survivor study. *Journal of Clinical Oncology, 22*, 999–1006. doi:10.1200/JCO.2004.06.148

CHAPTER 5

CAM THERAPY USE BY SITE

WHAT IS THE USE OF CAM BY CANCER SITE?

The use of CAM therapies in the United States crosses over disease types, practice settings, age, gender, and cultural and ethnic groups. A large survey of cancer survivors showed that patients with metastatic disease use CAM at higher rates than survivors with local disease. Breast cancer, ovarian cancer, and non-Hodgkin lymphoma survivors were the most likely to use CAM. Finally, this survey showed that the most common CAM therapies used by survivors were similar to ones used by people without cancer: spiritual practices, relaxation methods, and dietary supplements.

Common themes exist among patients considering CAM for cancer prevention, cancer treatment, and related symptoms:

- Many patients want to be involved in the planning and delivery of their care.
- Patients seek information from various sources and spend out-of-pocket dollars on health and wellness.
- Many patients use CAM without the knowledge of their healthcare providers.
- Safe and effective CAM therapies are available for some conditions.
- CAM studies need to fill the gaps between what is shown to be safe and effective in well-designed studies.

Are there examples of CAM therapies that are safe and effective for the treatment of cancer?

Several therapies now used for cancer treatment were once considered CAM. The reason for this is that they originated from the field of natural products or botanicals. The most notable example is Taxol®, which is a cancer drug made from a natural product that comes from the *Taxus baccata* tree.

Are CAM therapies available for the treatment of my cancer?

This section focuses on the CAM therapies that have been studied as well as what is under study for the following cancers: breast, colon and rectal, lung, lymphoma, ovarian, and prostate. For these cancers, studies have shown that CAM use is common and growing. People with cancer use CAM to boost the immune system, prevent cancer, slow the progression of the cancer, prevent recurrence, improve symptoms, and provide a greater sense of control over the disease. The most common therapies used are nutrition/diet, vitamins and minerals, teas, and complex natural products. The popular dietary changes are in line with current nutritional suggestions for good health (such as decreasing meat and fat intake, decreasing alcohol intake, and increasing intake of cruciferous fruits and vegetables). Many people who make dietary changes also reported using herbal and vitamin supplements.

Is information available on CAM therapies not covered in this section?

CAM clinical trials are added daily to the National Cancer Institute clinical trials database for the tumors discussed in this section as well as for adreno-cortical, bladder, endometrial, esophageal, head and neck, and pancreatic cancers, leukemia, melanoma, mesothelioma, and neuroendocrine skin cancer (see Resources).

BREAST CANCER

What is the role of CAM in chemoprevention and treatment of breast cancer?

CAM therapies that may prevent breast cancer recurrence either in the laboratory or in studies are CoQ10, curcumin, diindolylmethane, flaxseed lignans, green tea, indole-3-carbonol, L-glutamine, melatonin, omega-3 fatty acids, proanthocyanidins, vitamin D, and vitamin E.

CAM therapies that women with breast cancer should avoid are the herbal tonics Flor-Essence and Essiac, as these products may promote human breast cancer cell growth. Other supplements that may promote breast cancer cell growth are soy and soy products, red clover, licorice, dong quai, alfalfa extracts, ginkgo, ginseng, and pomegranate.

What CAM therapies are currently under study for chemoprevention and treatment of breast cancer?

- Examples for chemoprevention: vitamin D_3, soy protein, soy isoflavones, green tea, sulforaphane in broccoli sprout extract, cholecalciferol, natural flaxseed lignans, IH636 grape seed proanthocyanidin extract, freeze-dried table grape powder
- Examples for treatment: diindolylmethane, icaritin, soy isoflavones

COLON AND RECTAL CANCERS

What is the role of CAM in chemoprevention and treatment of colon and rectal cancers?

Increased physical activity is a lifestyle change that may reduce the risk of death for a patient who has been treated for colon cancer. Increased consumption of fiber and fish may help to protect against the disease.

CAM therapies that may be helpful in treating colon and rectal cancers either in the laboratory or in studies are aged garlic extract, anthocyanidins (extracts from berries), arabinogalactans (polysaccharides from the larch tree), curcumin, flaxseed, folic acid, green tea, indole-3-carbinol, L-glutamine, melatonin, mushroom extracts (maitake, reishi, *Cordyceps*), omega-3 fatty acids, quercetin, resveratrol, vitamin D and calcium, and vitamin E succinate (specific form of vitamin E).

What CAM therapies are currently under study for chemoprevention and treatment of colon and rectal cancers?

- Examples for chemoprevention: selenium and vitamin E for the prevention of polyps, inositol for colitis-associated dysplasia, cruciferous vegetables
- Examples for treatment: curcumin with gemcitabine and celecoxib, vitamin D_3, PHY906, high-dose vitamin D, green tea extract, green tea extract with milk thistle, fish oil

LUNG CANCER

What is the role of CAM in chemoprevention and treatment of lung cancer?

Decreasing or eliminating cigarette smoking may prevent or halt the development of some types of lung cancer. Methods to aid in quitting smoking include combining conventional nicotine aids (gum and patch) with acupuncture, behavioral modification, and supplements (vitamin C, thioglycerol, and an Indian tobacco plant called *Lobelia inflata*).

Studies show that beta-carotene may increase the risk of lung cancer in past or current smokers.

CAM therapies that may be helpful in promoting better health in those with lung cancer include protein-rich diets and those high in green leafy vegetables and fresh fruits.

CAM therapies that may be helpful in treating non-small cell lung cancer either in the laboratory or in studies are antioxidants (flavonoids, vitamin E, selenium, and vitamin C), ashwagandha along with paclitaxel, astragalus along with cisplatin or carboplatin, curcumin, green tea, melatonin, omega-3 fatty acids, and silymarin (flavonoid found in milk thistle).

What CAM therapies are currently under study for chemoprevention and treatment of lung cancer?

• Examples for chemoprevention: melatonin, vitamin D_3, green tea for bronchial dysplasia
• Examples for treatment: selected vegetable and herb mix (specialized formula of nontoxic botanicals containing known anticancer and/or immune-enhancing components), phytotherapy (in the form of blueberry powder), flaxseed, beta-glucan extracted from baker's yeast

LYMPHOMA

What is the role of CAM in chemoprevention and treatment of lymphoma?

Increased physical activity and avoiding obesity are lifestyle changes that may prevent the development of non-Hodgkin lymphoma. CAM interventions such as exercise and nutrition (maintaining healthy weight, increasing fruits and vegetables) are important.

CAM therapies that may be helpful in treating lymphoma either in the laboratory or in studies are genistein, green tea, L-carnitine, melatonin, mistletoe, and phytochemicals.

CAM therapies that should be avoided in patients with lymphoma are astragalus and long-term use of immune-stimulating mushrooms (shiitake, maitake, and fungus *Coriolus versicolor*). Astragalus has increased the production of white blood cells in the lab and may increase the growth of lymphoma.

What CAM therapies are currently under study for chemoprevention and treatment of lymphoma?

- Example for chemoprevention: vitamin D_3
- Examples for treatment: Se-methyl-seleno-L-cysteine with combination chemotherapy, intravenous vitamin C, nano-curcumin and resveratrol (either alone or in combination)

OVARIAN CANCER

What is the role of CAM in chemoprevention and treatment of ovarian cancer?

Nutrition and dietary factors are important in the development of ovarian cancer. Studies show that countries with populations that consume a higher amount of fat have higher rates of ovarian cancer. The hormones in milk products are being studied as a potential cause. The suggestion is to drink hormone-free or organic dairy products when possible.

Drinking green and black tea lowers the risk of developing ovarian cancer. One cup of tea per day reduced the risk by 24%, drinking two cups a day decreased the risk by 40%.

CAM therapies that may be helpful in the treatment of ovarian cancer are antioxidants (such as vitamins C and E, beta-carotene, and CoQ10), curcumin, ginkgo biloba, green tea, melatonin, mushroom polysaccharides (in *Agaricus blazei Murill* Kyowa), quercetin, soy, and vitamins A and D.

What CAM therapies are currently under study for chemoprevention and treatment of ovarian cancer?

- Examples for chemoprevention: No CAM therapies were under study at the time of printing.
- Examples for treatment: No CAM therapies were under study at the time of printing.

PROSTATE CANCER

What is the role of CAM in chemoprevention and treatment of prostate cancer?

The use of nutrition in the chemoprevention of prostate cancer began when studies showed that diet is related to a lower risk of cancer development. Scientists discovered that molecules are present in food that may kill or slow the growth of prostate cancer cells in the lab. Some examples are vitamin E, selenium, lycopene, and green tea.

Some studies have looked at CAM therapies for the treatment of prostate cancer. These include soy protein isolate, pomegranate extract, lycopene, vitamin D, vitamin E, selenium, green catechin extract, and prostate health cocktail (vitamin D_3, vitamin E, selenium, green tea extract, saw palmetto, lycopene, and soy derivatives).

What CAM therapies are currently under study for chemoprevention and treatment of prostate cancer?

• Examples for chemoprevention: soy protein, selenium, polyphenon E, vitamin E, lycopene
• Examples for treatment: muscadine grape skin extract, vitamin D and soy, prostate health cocktail (see previous), green tea, selenomethionine, high-dose vitamin C, and genistein

BIBLIOGRAPHY

Introduction

American Cancer Society. (2011). Complementary and alternative methods for cancer management. Retrieved from http://www.cancer.org/Treatment/TreatmentsandSideEffects/ComplementaryandAlternativeMedicine

Bristol-Myers Squibb. (2011). *Taxol® (paclitaxel) injection* [Package insert]. Retrieved from http://packageinserts.bms.com/pi/pi_taxol.pdf

Gansler, T., Kaw, C., Crammer, C., & Smith, T. (2008). A population-based study of prevalence of complementary methods use by cancer survivors: A report from the American Cancer Society's studies of cancer survivors. *Cancer, 113,* 1048–1057. doi:10.1002/cncr.23659

Lee, C.O. (2009). Complementary and integrative therapies. In B.H. Gobel, S. Triest-Robertson, & W.H. Vogel (Eds.), *Advanced oncology nursing certification review and resource manual* (pp. 305–327). Pittsburgh, PA: Oncology Nursing Society.

Breast Cancer

Alschuler, L., & Gazella, K.A. (2007). Breast cancer. In *Alternative Medicine Magazine's definitive guide to cancer: An integrated approach to prevention, treatment, and healing* (2nd ed., pp. 320–332). Berkeley, CA: Celestial Arts.

Mumber, M.P. (Ed.). (2006). *Integrative oncology: Principles and practice.* Abingdon, Oxon, UK: Taylor & Francis.

National Cancer Institute. (2011). Clinical trials. Retrieved from http://www.cancer.gov/clinicaltrials

Colon and Rectal Cancers

Alschuler, L., & Gazella, K.A. (2007). Colon cancer. In *Alternative Medicine Magazine's definitive guide to cancer: An integrated approach to prevention, treatment, and healing* (2nd ed., pp. 338–345). Berkeley, CA: Celestial Arts.

Lieberman, D.A., Prindiville, S., Weiss, D.G., & Willett, W. (2003). Risk factors for advanced colonic neoplasia and hyperplastic polyps in asymptomatic individuals. *JAMA, 290,* 2959–2967. doi:10.1001/jama.290.22.2959

Meyerhardt, J.A., Giovannucci, E.L., Holmes, M.D., Chan, A.T., Chan, J.A., Colditz, G.A., & Fuchs, C.S. (2006). Physical activity and survival after colorectal cancer diagnosis. *Journal of Clinical Oncology, 24,* 3527–3534. doi:10.1200/JCO.2006.06.0855

National Cancer Institute. (2011). Clinical trials. Retrieved from http://www.cancer.gov/clinicaltrials

Lung Cancer

Alschuler, L., & Gazella, K.A. (2007). Lung cancer. In *Alternative Medicine Magazine's definitive guide to cancer: An integrated approach to prevention, treatment, and healing* (2nd ed., pp. 376–381). Berkeley, CA: Celestial Arts.

National Cancer Institute. (2011). Cancer CAM clinical trials. Retrieved from http://www.cancer.gov/clinicaltrials/search/results?protocolsearchid=6572492

Patel, J.D., Bach, P.B., & Kris, M.G. (2004). Lung cancer in US women: A contemporary epidemic. *JAMA, 291,* 1763–1768. doi:10.1001/jama.291.14.1763

Lymphoma

Alschuler, L., & Gazella, K.A. (2007). Leukemia, lymphoma, and myeloma. In *Alternative Medicine Magazine's definitive guide to cancer: An integrated approach to prevention, treatment, and healing* (2nd ed., pp. 356–369). Berkeley, CA: Celestial Arts.

National Cancer Institute. (2011). Clinical trials. Retrieved from http://www.cancer.gov/clinicaltrials

Pan, S.Y., Mao, Y., & Ugnat, A.M. (2005). Physical activity, obesity, energy intake, and the risk of non-Hodgkin's lymphoma: A population-based case-control study. *American Journal of Epidemiology, 162,* 1162–1173. doi:10.1093/aje/kwi312

Ovarian Cancer

Alschuler, L., & Gazella, K.A. (2007). Ovarian cancer. In *Alternative Medicine Magazine's definitive guide to cancer: An integrated approach to prevention, treatment, and healing* (2nd ed., pp. 385–390). Berkeley, CA: Celestial Arts.

Ganmaa, D., & Sato, A. (2005). The possible role of female sex hormones in milk from pregnant cows in the development of breast, ovarian, and corpus uteri cancers. *Medical Hypotheses, 65,* 1028–1037. doi:10.1016/j.mehy.2005.06.026

Larsson, S.C., & Wolk, A. (2005). Tea consumption and ovarian cancer risk in a population-based cohort. *Archives of Internal Medicine, 165,* 2683–2686. doi:10.1001/archinte.165.22.2683

National Cancer Institute. (2011). Clinical trials. Retrieved from http://www.cancer.gov/clinicaltrials

Prostate Cancer

Eng, J., Ramsum, D., Verhoef, M., Guns, E., Davison, J., & Gallagher, R. (2003). A population-based survey of complementary and alternative medicine use in men recently diagnosed with prostate cancer. *Integrative Cancer Therapies, 2,* 212–216. doi:10.1177/1534735403256207

Chan, J.M., Elkin, E.P., Silva, S.J., Broering, J.M., Latini, D.M., & Carroll, P.R. (2005). Total and specific complementary and alternative medicine use in a large cohort of men with prostate cancer. *Urology, 66,* 1223–1228. doi:10.1016/j.urology.2005.06.003

National Cancer Institute. (2011). Clinical trials. Retrieved from http://www.cancer.gov/clinicaltrials

Wilkinson, S., Farrelly, S., Low, J., Chakraborty, A., Williams, R., & Wilkinson, S. (2008). The use of complementary therapy by men with prostate cancer in the UK. *European Journal of Cancer Care, 17,* 492–499. doi:10.1111/j.1365-2354.2007.00904.x

CHAPTER 6

HEALTHY LIVING

INTRODUCTION

As previously discussed, people seek out natural products for a variety of reasons, including treating disease, maintaining health, and promoting wellness. Interest in the use of natural supplements for cancer prevention is growing. The National Center for Complementary and Alternative Medicine (NCCAM) considers natural products as dietary supplements and includes vitamins, minerals, probiotics, and herbal medicines. The National Cancer Institute's Office of Cancer Complementary and Alternative Medicine (OCCAM) uses the term *nutritional therapeutics* to describe supplements used as cancer-preventing agents. These include a variety of nutrients, non-nutrients, and bioactive food components for cancer prevention.

> *"He that takes medicine and neglects diet wastes the skills of the physician."*
> —Chinese proverb

> *"To eat is a necessity, but to eat intelligently is an art."*
> —La Rochefoucauld

What are the kinds of cancer prevention?

- Primary—to decrease the risk of developing cancer
- Secondary—early screening to identify cancer in the precancerous or early stage

- Tertiary—prevention of recurrence, metastasis, or a secondary cancer

Are there natural products that I can take to prevent cancer?

No natural products have been established for primary and tertiary cancer prevention. Some research suggests that various vitamins, minerals, and dietary components reduce the risk of developing specific cancers. Currently no recommendations exist. Based on current research, guidelines advise against the use of dietary supplements for cancer prevention. Research is ongoing.

What is being researched?

Refer to Chapter 3 for information on vitamins and supplements. Other examples include the following.

Green Tea

Some studies suggest that green tea may reduce the risk of upper gastrointestinal tract, lung, liver, and breast cancers. Studies are starting to look at potential benefit in oral, skin, cervical, and prostate cancer prevention. Clinical trials are ongoing on the use of green tea for breast cancer prevention (see www.clinicaltrials.gov, trials NCT00917735 and NCT00676793).

Soy

Soy contains isoflavones, which are of interest for cancer prevention because of the phytoestrogenic and antioxidant effects. One study suggests that soy may decrease tumor progression in patients with low-grade prostate cancer, but research results have been conflicting.

Curcumin

Curcumin is of particular interest in cancer prevention for its antioxidant and anti-inflammatory effects. It is poorly absorbed, and most of the current research has focused on colorectal cancer prevention because of the direct contact with the colonic mucosa.

Probiotics

Probiotics are live microorganisms found in dietary supplements and fermented food such as yogurt and kefir. They are thought to offer cancer prevention benefits for the gastrointestinal tract by making changes in the gut that control the growth of harmful bacteria and improve immune function. More research is needed to understand the way that probiotics may work in cancer prevention.

My friends have recommended that I "detoxify." What is detoxification?

Our digestive system (also known as our gastrointestinal, or GI, tract) has exposure to and with the "outside" world. It takes about three days to complete the process of turning food into energy and eliminating any toxins that might have been associated with food or beverage intake. Keeping this system running smoothly is extremely important to avoid digestive system illnesses and diseases. There are cancers that are directly and indirectly associated with toxins. You can read more about these associations at the Web sites of the American Cancer Society (www.cancer.org) and the National Cancer Institute (www.cancer.gov), as well as others (see Resources).

How can I detoxify? What herbs or natural products should I take to detoxify?

The best way to begin to detoxify is to stop putting the "toxic" foods or products into your body. A forced cleanse using special products can be very difficult for your body to tolerate. Gradual elimination of toxic or unhealthy foods and products will not overwork a body that already has a lot to do. Toxins in the body are believed to stimulate an inflammatory reaction, one of three factors thought to promote the development of cancer or recurrence of cancer. (The three factors are inflammation, oxidative stress, and altered immune response.) Following is the ultimate to-do list for health and wellness:

- Eliminate refined sugar (see "Some Sweet Deceptions").
- Eliminate products that contain enriched flour (see "Wheat-Free Cooking").
- Eliminate processed foods (if you have eliminated refined sugar and enriched flour, you have eliminated many processed foods).
- Buy organic and locally grown produce whenever possible.
- Check out the Environmental Working Group's "Dirty Dozen" at www.foodnews.org. They list the fresh fruits and vegetables that retain the highest and lowest amounts of pesticides. It can guide you when deciding what to buy organic and when you can opt for conventionally grown produce.
- Wash fruits and vegetables well. You can use pesticide-removing spray from the health food store or apple cider vinegar.
- Avoid or drastically reduce intake of fish known to contain mercury: swordfish, tuna, shark, and marlin.

- Avoid or drastically reduce intake of alcoholic beverages.
- Chew food well to aid digestion and avoid the buildup of half-digested food toxins in the stomach.
- Choose detoxifying foods such as cruciferous vegetables (brussels sprouts, broccoli, cauliflower, cabbage, kale, and others—but increase the use of these vegetables gradually to avoid gas pains, especially if you have irritable bowel syndrome or other stomach or bowel conditions), onions, omega-3 eggs (limit consumption), sea vegetables, fish, legumes, and whey protein.
- Drink six to eight glasses of safe water (water from home filtering systems or spring water). Caffeine-free herbal teas and juice count toward this intake.
- Consider filtering shower and bath water to decrease exposure to contaminants.
- Open your windows. It has been estimated that airtight buildings have two to five times the pollutants of outdoor air (and according to the U.S. Environmental Protection Agency, this number can be up to 100 times). This may not be the case in some industrial cities or areas. Use caution if you have seasonal allergies.
- Avoid using air fresheners; instead, use plants, which naturally absorb pollutants.
- Use cleaning products containing less toxic ingredients.
- Use household products (carpets, paint, etc.) that do not release toxic compounds.
- Minimize dry cleaning clothing with perchloroethylene (suspected to be a carcinogen).
- Wash all clothes before wearing.
- Test your place of residence for radon.

- Eliminate any mold in your home. Tests kits for mold are available at home improvement and building product stores and online.
- Avoid or minimize the use of pesticides indoors (for example, some flea products for pets).
- Avoid or minimize the use of yard and lawn chemicals.

Make small changes over time. It can be overwhelming to try to make all of these changes within a short time frame. For example:

- Week 1—Take time to chew food well.
- Week 2—Gradually eliminate all refined sugar from your diet according to the following schedule. (Cravings will stop in about three days after eliminating all sugar and processed foods.)
  - Sunday and Monday: breakfast
  - Tuesday and Wednesday: breakfast and snacks
  - Thursday and Friday: breakfast, snacks, and lunch
  - Saturday: breakfast, snacks, lunch, and dinner
- Week 3—Continue with the previous changes, and eliminate all "enriched" flour
- Week 4—Continue with the previous changes, and eliminate any/all remaining processed foods.
- Week 5—Continue with the previous changes, and buy organic and wash produce thoroughly.
- Week 6—Continue with the previous changes, and avoid mercury-containing fish.
- Week 7—Continue with the previous changes, and avoid or minimize alcohol consumption.

A final "ingredient" is your wellness plan. It should be individualized to meet your needs and any restrictions you might have. Please be very careful to have a properly credentialed professional assist you with this plan. Keep it simple and appropriate for your health history, and be consistent.

I start nutrition and exercise programs but then stop after a few weeks. How do I keep myself going?

Keep a nutrition and fitness journal. Significant research has shown that those who keep nutrition and activity journals are more successful at reaching and maintaining goals. You will be able to track your milestones. Remember that making a notation that you ate a bowl of cereal does not tell you anything—you also need to record the serving portion (½ cup, ¾ cup), the kind of milk, and other details. You can follow this suggested format for a nutrition/activity/symptom journal:

Date:
Food: Record what time you ate, if you ate, what you ate, and how much you ate. • Breakfast: • Snack: • Lunch: • Snack: • Dinner: • Snack:
Exercise: What kind? How much or how long?
Comments: Record your mood, sleep, comments regarding foods that you may identify as "not agreeing" with you, etc.

I have read that inflammation is seen in chronic illnesses, including cancer. How do I decrease inflammation in my body?

Begin by stabilizing your blood sugar by avoiding the foods described earlier in this chapter, such as refined sugar, enriched flour, alcohol, and processed foods. Concentrate on eating healthy food that has a balance of complex carbohydrates and protein. See "MyPlate," below.

I was told there are two kinds of carbohydrates: simple and complex. What is the difference?

Simply said, simple carbohydrates are broken down into glucose faster than complex carbohydrates. Simple carbohydrates include bread, pasta, baked goods, fruits that contain high amounts of natural sugars, and starchy vegetables (such as corn and peas). Complex carbohydrates are broken down more slowly than simple carbohydrates; fruits and vegetables and whole grains fall into this category.

In 2011, the U.S. Department of Agriculture released a new model for building a healthy plate that is in line with the 2010 dietary guidelines (see www .dietaryguidelines.gov). The new icon (see left) emphasizes the fruit, vegetable, grain, protein, and dairy food groups. More information about MyPlate, along with healthy meal ideas, recipes, and a food and exercise tracker, is available at www.choosemyplate .gov.

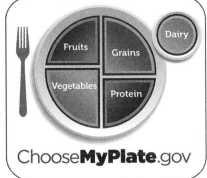
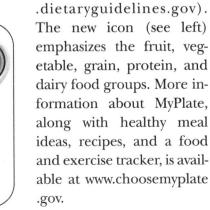

I like to cook, but it seems like I will have to change everything I do—and the way I do it!

You can still use your personal recipes, but you may need to change a few ingredients or make some modifications in the preparation. For example, you will want to avoid deep frying, but you can try "oven frying" or sautéing. Visit your local health food store or bookstore to look at the cookbooks for ideas. Many communities now provide healthy cooking classes through a cooperative extension program or local healthcare organizations. Healthy versions of recipes also can be found on the Internet

SOME SWEET DECEPTIONS

In the world of sweeteners, the term *natural* may be used to describe any nutritive sweetener, in other words, those that contain calories. This includes all forms of sugar. Many people misinterpret this as "unrefined" or even "nutritious." Many "natural" sweeteners are highly processed and do not make any significant contribution to the diet other than calories.

Some people do not care what form their sweetener takes, whereas others are willing to pay a high price for what they believe to be a less processed, more natural product. We are often deceived by the promise of "no sugar added," as food labels are permitted to make this claim as long as the common sugar extracted from cane or beets is absent. This is a very narrow interpretation of the word *sugar*.

There are many different kinds of sugar (such as glucose, fructose, sucrose, maltose, dextrose, lactose, galactose, and levulose). All nutritive sweeteners, no matter what the name, contain one or more of these sugars.

When you are trying to determine the total sugar content of a food, keep in mind that food manufacturers want their sugar content to be less obvious and often add several different sugars to their product. This means that instead of showing up as one item near the top of the ingredient list, the sweeteners are sprinkled throughout.

The Way Sugars Show Up on a Label		
• Barley malt	• Glucose syrup	• Maple syrup
• Brown sugar	• High fructose	• Molasses
• Corn sweetener	• Honey	• Raw sugar
• Corn syrup	• Invert sugar	• Rice syrup
• Date sugar	• Lactose	• Sorbitol
• Demerara sugar	• Levulose	• Sucrose
• Dextrose	• Malted grain	• Sugar
• Fructose	syrups	• Turbinado sugar
• Fruit sugar	• Maltose	• Xylitol
	• Mannitol	

Note. Used with permission from Integrative Care, Albany, NY.

WHEAT-FREE COOKING (AVOIDING THE USE OF "ENRICHED" FLOUR)

People with sensitivities to wheat can experiment with some alternatives to traditional flour. Non-wheat flours have different consistencies and properties and cannot be directly substituted for wheat flour. Suggestions include the following.

• For thickening gravies and sauces, replace wheat flour with an equal amount of rice or corn flour. You may also use arrowroot, cornstarch, or potato starch by decreasing the amount of wheat flour you would use by half.

• Prepare crumb coatings by crushing corn tacos, rice, rye crackers, or appropriate cereals.

- When baking without wheat, the baked goods will be dense and heavy because they lack gluten, which is needed for rising. However, some baked goods can be made quite successfully without wheat. Examples include those made using baking powder, baking soda, and/or eggs for leavening. If you are unable to locate recipes, try using the following conversions when baking: To replace 1 cup of wheat flour in baked goods, use
  - 1 cup corn flour
  - ¾ cup corn meal
  - ⅞ cup (brown) rice flour
  - ⅞ cup buckwheat flour
  - 1½ cups rye flour
  - ⅝ cup potato flour
  - ½ cup barley flour
  - ½ cup ground nuts or seeds
  - 1½ cup ground oats or oat flour.
- Choose recipes that use only small amounts of flour, like sponge cake, brownies, or angel food cakes. You will probably obtain the best results when using a combination of the ingredients noted above. Wheat-free baked goods tend to crumble easily; therefore, it is better to make small-size products (such as biscuits and rolls instead of breads and muffins, and cupcakes instead of cakes).
- You will probably have to make adjustments in the amount of liquids—you will usually need more.
- You will probably have to make adjustments in the amount of shortening—you will usually need less.
- To help improve the texture of your baked goods, you may want to add an extra ½ teaspoon baking powder per cup of flour.
- Wheat-free products should be baked at a lower temperature.

ADDITIONAL RESOURCES

- *The Cancer-Fighting Kitchen: Nourishing, Big-Flavor Recipes for Cancer Treatment and Recovery*, by Rebecca Katz with Mat Edelson, 2009, New York, NY: Ten Speed Press.
- *Cookies for Kids' Cancer: Best Bake Sale Cookbook*, by Gretchen Holt-Witt and Lucy Schaeffer, 2011, Hoboken, NJ: John Wiley and Sons.
- *Eating Well Through Cancer: Easy Recipes and Recommendations During and After Treatment*, by Holly Clegg and Gerald Miletello, 2006, Memphis, TN: Wimmer Companies.
- *Nutrition and Cancer: Practical Tips and Tasty Recipes for Survivors*, by Sandra L. Luthringer and Valerie J. Kogut, 2011, Pittsburgh, PA: Hygeia Media.
- *What to Eat During Cancer Treatment: 100 Great-Tasting, Family-Friendly Recipes to Help You Cope*, by Jeanne Besser, Kristina Ratley, Sheri Knecht and Michele Szafranski, 2009, Atlanta, GA: American Cancer Society.

FOR MORE INFORMATION

AMERICAN BOTANICAL COUNCIL

- Commission E Monographs: http://cms.herbalgram .org/commissione/index.html
- HerbClip™ Online: http://cms.herbalgram.org/ herbclip/index.html
- HerbMedPro(membershipfee):http://cms.herbalgram .org/herbmedpro/overview.html
- Monographs: http://abc.herbalgram.org/site/Page Server?pagename=Monographs

AMERICAN CANCER SOCIETY

- ComplementaryandAlternativeTherapies:www.cancer .org/docroot/ETO/ETO_5.asp?sitearea=ETO
- Nutrition for Children with Cancer: www.cancer.org/ docroot/MBC/MBC_6_1_nutrition_for_children_ with_cancer.asp
- Nutrition for the Person With Cancer: www.cancer .org/docroot/MBC/MBC_6.asp?sitearea=ETO

CANCER CENTERS WITH CAM/INTEGRATIVE PROGRAMS

- ArizonaCenterforIntegrativeMedicine:http://integrative medicine.arizona.edu

- Duke Integrative Medicine: www.dukeintegrative medicine.org
- George Washington Center for Integrative Medicine: www.integrativemedicinedc.com
- Integrative Medicine Service at Memorial Sloan-Kettering Cancer Center: www.mskcc.org/mskcc/html/1979.cfm
- Johns Hopkins Center for Complementary and Alternative Medicine: www.hopkinsmedicine.org/CAM
- Osher Clinical Center for Complementary and Integrative Medical Therapies: www.brighamandwomens.org/medicine/oshercenter
- Rosenthal Center for Complementary and Alternative Medicine: www.rosenthal.hs.columbia.edu
- Stanford Center for Integrative Medicine: Clinical Services for Mind and Body: http://stanfordhospital.org/clinicsmedServices/clinics/complementary Medicine
- University of Pittsburgh Center for Integrative Medicine: www.upmc.com/Services/integrative-medicine/Pages/default.aspx
- University of Texas MD Anderson Cancer Center Complementary/Integrative Medicine Education Resources: www.mdanderson.org/education-and-research/resources-for-professionals/clinical-tools-and-resources/cimer/index.html
- Vanderbilt Center for Integrative Medicine: www.vanderbilthealth.com/integrativehealth

DATABASES (FREE)

- HerbMed® Top 20 Herbs in the U.S. market: www.herbmed.org/#param.wapp?sw_page=top20

- Medline Plus: www.nlm.nih.gov/medlineplus/com plementaryandalternativemedicine.html
- National Institutes of Health Office of Dietary Supplements Dietary Supplement Label Database: http:// ods.od.nih.gov/Health_Information/Dietary_Supplement_Ingredient_and_Labeling_Databases .aspx

DATABASES (FOR-FEE)

- HerbMedPro® pay-per-day or multisite user licenses: www.herbmed.org/#param.wapp?sw_page= subscriptions
- Natural Standard
  - Patient Handouts: Foods, Herbs and Supplements: http://naturalstandard.com/tools/handouts/hsf/a/
  - Patient Handouts: Health and Wellness: http:// naturalstandard.com/tools/handouts/hw/A/
- Natural Medicines Comprehensive Database
  - Clinical Management Series and Special Reports: http://naturaldatabase.therapeuticresearch .com/nd/ClinicalMngt.aspx?cs=&s=ND
  - Consumer Version: http://naturaldatabaseconsumer .therapeuticresearch.com/home.aspx?cs=&s=NDC

PEDIATRIC-SPECIFIC RESOURCES

- CAM Wellness Center: http://integrativetherapies .columbia.edu
- Carol Ann's Library Book Catalogue: http://integra tivetherapies.columbia.edu/book_catalog.html
- Summary of Medical Literature for CAM in Children with Cancer: http://integrativetherapies.columbia .edu/research/SumMLit.html

- Surveys on CAM use in pediatric oncology population: http://integrativetherapies.columbia.edu/research/surv.html

U.S. FEDERAL GOVERNMENT

Agency for Healthcare Research and Quality

- Cancer Prevention: Vitamin Supplements: www.ahrq.gov/clinic/uspstf/uspsvita.htm
- Meditation Practices for Health: State of the Research: www.ahrq.gov/downloads/pub/evidence/pdf/meditation/medit.pdf
- Melatonin: Sleep Disorders: www.ahrq.gov/news/press/pr2004/melatnpr.htm

U.S. Department of Agriculture

- Food and Nutrition Information Center: http://fnic.nal.usda.gov/nal_display/index.php?tax_level=1&info_center=4

U.S. Department of Health and Human Services

- White House Commission on Complementary and Alternative Medicine Policy: www.whccamp.hhs.gov/finalreport.html

U.S. Federal Trade Commission

- Consumer Education on Diet, Health, and Fitness: www.ftc.gov/bcp/menus/consumer/health.shtm
- Operation False Cure: www.ftc.gov/bcp/edu/microsites/curious/share.shtml

U.S. Food and Drug Administration

- Buying Medicines and Medical Products Online: www.fda.gov/ForConsumers/ProtectYourSelf/default.htm

- Center for Food Safety and Applied Nutrition: Dietary Supplements: www.fda.gov/Food/Dietary Supplements/default.htm
- Tips for Older Dietary Supplement Users: www.fda .gov/Food/DietarySupplements/ConsumerInform ation/ucm110493.htm
- Tips for the Savvy Supplement User: Making Informed Decisions and Evaluating Information: www .fda.gov/Food/DietarySupplements/Consumer Information/ucm110567.htm

U.S. National Institutes of Health

- National Institute on Aging: www.nia.nih.gov
- NIHSeniorHealth: http://nihseniorhealth.gov
- National Institute of Arthritis and Musculoskeletal and Skin Diseases: Phytoestrogens and Bone Health: www.niams.nih.gov/Health_Info/Bone/Osteo porosis/Menopause/default.asp
- National Library of Medicine: www.nlm.nih.gov
  - CAM on PubMed®: http://nccam.nih.gov/ research/camonpubmed
  - Dietary Supplements Labels Database: http:// dietarysupplements.nlm.nih.gov/dietary
  - DIRLINE: http://dirline.nlm.nih.gov
  - MedlinePlus Complementary and Alternative Medicine Page: www.nlm.nih.gov/medlineplus/ complementaryandalternativemedicine.html
  - MedlinePlus Drugs, Supplements and Herbal Information: www.nlm.nih.gov/medlineplus/ druginformation.html
  - MedlinePlus Herbal Medicine Page: www.nlm.nih .gov/medlineplus/herbalmedicine.html
  - National Lirbary of Medicine FAQs: Dietary Supplements, Complementary or Alternative Medicincs: www.nlm.nih.gov/scrviccs/dietsup.html

- National Cancer Institute: www.cancer.gov
  - Cancer Information Service: http://cis.nci.nih.gov
  - Fact Sheets: www.nci.nih.gov/cancertopics/factsheet
  - Office of Cancer Complementary and Alternative Medicine: www.cancer.gov/cam
  - PDQ® Cancer Information Summaries: Complementary and Alternative Medicine: www.cancer.gov/cancertopics/pdq/cam
  - PDQ® Cancer Information Summaries: Supportive and Palliative Care (Coping With Cancer): www.cancer.gov/cancertopics/pdq/supportivecare
- National Center for Complementary and Alternative Medicine: http://nccam.nih.gov/health
  - Herbs at a Glance: http://nccam.nih.gov/health/herbsataglance.htm
- Office of Dietary Supplements (General): http://ods.od.nih.gov/index.aspx
  - Annual Bibliographies of Significant Advances in Dietary Supplement Research: http://ods.od.nih.gov/Research/Annual_Bibliographies.aspx
  - Botanical Dietary Supplements: Background Information: http://ods.od.nih.gov/factsheets/botanicalbackground.asp
  - Botanical Research Centers Program: http://ods.od.nih.gov/Research/Dietary_Supplement_Research_Centers.aspx
  - Computer Access to Research on Dietary SupplementsDatabase:http://ods.od.nih.gov/Research/CARDS_Database.aspx
  - Dietary Supplement Ingredient Database: http://dietarysupplementdatabase.usda.nih.gov
  - Fact Sheets and Background Information: http://ods.od.nih.gov/Health_Information/Information_About_Individual_Dietary_Supplements.aspx

– Frequently Asked Questions: http://ods.od.nih .gov/Health_Information/ODS_Frequently_ Asked_Questions.aspx
International Bibliographic Information on Dietary Supplements Database: http://ods.od.nih .gov/Health_Information/IBIDS.aspx

Substance Abuse and Mental Health Services Administration

- Alternative Approaches to Mental Health Care: http://mentalhealth.samhsa.gov/publications/ allpubs/KEN98-0044/default.asp